NOV 1 6 2017

IT HAPPENED TO ME

Series Editor: Arlene Hirschfelder

Books in the It Happened to Me series are designed for inquisitive teens digging for answers about certain illnesses, social issues, or lifestyle interests. Whether you are deep into your teen years or just entering them, these books are gold mines of up-to-date information, riveting teen views, and great visuals to help you figure out stuff. Besides special boxes highlighting singular facts, each book is enhanced with the latest reading lists, websites, and an index. Perfect for browsing, there are loads of expert information by acclaimed writers to help parents, guardians, and librarians understand teen illness, tough situations, and lifestyle choices.

1. *Epilepsy: The Ultimate Teen Guide,* by Kathlyn Gay and Sean McGarrahan, 2002.
2. *Stress Relief: The Ultimate Teen Guide,* by Mark Powell, 2002.
3. *Learning Disabilities: The Ultimate Teen Guide,* by Penny Hutchins Paquette and Cheryl Gerson Tuttle, 2003.
4. *Making Sexual Decisions: The Ultimate Teen Guide,* by L. Kris Gowen, 2003.
5. *Asthma: The Ultimate Teen Guide,* by Penny Hutchins Paquette, 2003.
6. *Cultural Diversity—Conflicts and Challenges: The Ultimate Teen Guide,* by Kathlyn Gay, 2003.
7. *Diabetes: The Ultimate Teen Guide,* by Katherine J. Moran, 2004.
8. *When Will I Stop Hurting? Teens, Loss, and Grief: The Ultimate Teen Guide to Dealing with Grief,* by Ed Myers, 2004.
9. *Volunteering: The Ultimate Teen Guide,* by Kathlyn Gay, 2004.
10. *Organ Transplants—A Survival Guide for the Entire Family: The Ultimate Teen Guide,* by Tina P. Schwartz, 2005.
11. *Medications: The Ultimate Teen Guide,* by Cheryl Gerson Tuttle, 2005.
12. *Image and Identity—Becoming the Person You Are: The Ultimate Teen Guide,* by L. Kris Gowen and Molly C. McKenna, 2005.
13. *Apprenticeship: The Ultimate Teen Guide,* by Penny Hutchins Paquette, 2005.
14. *Cystic Fibrosis: The Ultimate Teen Guide,* by Melanie Ann Apel, 2006.
15. *Religion and Spirituality in America: The Ultimate Teen Guide,* by Kathlyn Gay, 2006.

49. *Chronic Illnesses, Syndromes, and Rare Disorders: The Ultimate Teen Guide,* by Marlene Targ Brill, 2016.
50. *Autism Spectrum Disorder: The Ultimate Teen Guide,* by Francis Tabone, 2016.
51. *Sexual Assault: The Ultimate Teen Guide,* by Olivia Ghafoerkhan, 2016.
52. *Epilepsy: The Ultimate Teen Guide, Second Edition,* by Kathlyn Gay, 2017.
53. *Sexual Decisions: The Ultimate Teen Guide, Second Edition,* by L. Kris Gowen, 2017.

SEXUAL DECISIONS

THE ULTIMATE TEEN GUIDE

SECOND EDITION

L. KRIS GOWEN

IT HAPPENED TO ME, NO. 53

ROWMAN & LITTLEFIELD
Lanham • Boulder • New York • London

Published by Rowman & Littlefield
A wholly owned subsidary of The Rowman & Littlefield Publishing Group, Inc.
4501 Forbes Boulevard, Suite 200, Lanham, Maryland 20706
www.rowman.com

Unit A, Whitacre Mews, 26-34 Stannary Street, London SE11 4AB

British Library Cataloguing in Publication Information Available

Library of Congress Cataloging-in-Publication Data

Names: Gowen, L. Kris, 1968– author.
Title: Sexual decisions : the ultimate teen guide / L. Kris Gowen.
Other titles: Making sexual decisions
Description: Second edition. | Lanham : Rowman & Littlefield, [2017] | Series: It happened
  to me ; no. 53 | Revision of: Making sexual decisions / L. Kris Gowen. 2003. | Includes
  bibliographical references and index.
Identifiers: LCCN 2016035811 (print) | LCCN 2016038656 (ebook) | ISBN 9781442277830
  (hardback : alk. paper) | ISBN 9781442277847 (electronic)
Subjects: LCSH: Sex instruction for teenagers. | Sex. | Teenagers—Sexual behavior.
Classification: LCC HQ35 .G68 2017 (print) | LCC HQ35 (ebook) | DDC 613.9071/2—dc23
LC record available at https://lccn.loc.gov/2016035811

Printed in the United States of America

To all the young people who helped shape this book, and to Molly McKenna, who continues to inspire me.

Contents

Acknowledgments

This book represents the ideas and experiences of many, in hopes of casting light on a hidden, complex, and emotional topic. Being a sexuality educator in the United States is no easy task, and it takes a lot of people coming together to make books like this possible. Special thanks to Arlene Hirschfelder, Stephen Ryan, and Rowman & Littlefield for giving me the chance to revise this book and allow difficult and important topics to make it to print; Carolyn Laub and Donnovan Somera, who mentored me in my early stages of being a sexuality educator and whose work at the Mid-Peninsula YWCA has impacted many young lives in northern California; Amy Nelson for her research support and incredible illustrations; Ieva and Malcolm Fraser for providing me with a safe place to work on my revisions; my amazing panel of reviewers, including Lauren Lichty, Megan Foster, Sofie Ofelia, Johanna Thomas, Mo Atkinson, Amy Evers, Carolina Main Mann, Ted Batt, and Edward Hashima; Nancy Brown and the doctors of the We Are Talking teen health website from the Palo Alto Medical Foundation, for providing questions and answers for this book; the many contributors of the Youth Speak Out sections; and to my mother and father for their continued support and love. Without all of your work and dedication to this project, it would not be on the shelves today.

Introduction

Fourteen years ago, I was asked to write this book and I thought I couldn't have been more excited. It was nothing short of a dream come true; I had been studying and teaching sexuality education for years, and this was my chance to put all my ideas onto paper for others to read. Then, when I was asked to write a revision, I got to relive the joy and challenge all over again! My ideas on the subject had changed, as had the landscape in which we live, love, and form relationships. A revision was indeed needed. True, some of the information has stayed the same, but a lot is different, because our situations are different. When it comes to sexuality and sexual health, we have more decisions to make than ever before.

Yet, despite all the changes and new things to consider, sexuality education remains rather lacking in our culture. Look at the examples. At school, you don't spend a lot of time in sex ed classes, if you even have a sex ed class at your school. Often, sexuality and sexual health are taught during a biology class or a health class, and sometimes only for a few days. Subjects like math and English get much more time and attention at every school in the United States. I'm not saying that math and English aren't important, but the amount of schooling you get in those two subjects as compared to sexuality and sexual health is astounding. And, in the end, you will probably need the information in a sex ed class more than, say, what you learn in trigonometry or while examining the works of Shakespeare.

Schools often don't spend a lot of time on sexuality education for many different reasons. They are faced with mandates that require them to focus on other subjects. Their state laws prevent them from addressing certain topics. They are concerned that angry parents will not appreciate what's being taught in the classes. Teachers aren't trained properly to teach sexuality education and therefore don't feel prepared to do so. The reasons are many and complicated both socially and politically.

Then there is getting sexuality education at home. Some family members do a great job talking to their children about sex. Unfortunately, many of my students have told me that quality sex education from family members doesn't happen very often. Most parents don't talk much about sex; again, there are many reasons this happens. Some parents want the schools to do it. Some are uncomfortable. Some believe they don't know enough to start a conversation. Some are afraid that it will

Abstinence Only versus Comprehensive Sex Ed

Although there are many different sexuality education curricula out there, sex ed in general can be divided into two types: comprehensive and abstinence until marriage. In comprehensive sexuality education, a student will learn about not only abstinence but also other forms of pregnancy and STD (sexually transmitted disease) prevention such as condoms and the pill. In an abstinence-until-marriage program, abstinence is the only method of pregnancy and STD prevention discussed; the idea is that a person must wait until marriage to have sex. I believe young people should have access to comprehensive sexuality education because it has shown to be more effective than abstinence until marriage.[a] I also believe that information should not be withheld from young people. In order to make sound decisions, people should have access to all the information they need to stay healthy, safe, and happy.

be awkward or that their children will reject them. Talking about sex takes courage from everyone! And, to be honest, not all young people want to hear about sex from their parents or close family members. So, a parent's idea of sex education may be something pretty simple and brief, like:

"Wait until you're married."
"Don't get pregnant" or "Don't get someone pregnant."
"Use a condom, please."

While these words of advice can be useful, young people need more information. In an ideal world, there would be many conversations about sex and a lot of different sex-related topics between a young person and a trusted adult. There wouldn't be just "the talk," and then sex is never spoken of again. But for the most part, it comes down to this: your school isn't giving you the answers you need—some of them may be, but not all for sure—and parents and other adults aren't clueing you in, either. So how important can sex education really be if no one is giving you the information you need? I mean, come on. Learning about sex only helps you learn about your body and your relationships with other people, and could possibly save your life. Are those things really *that* important? Of course they are.

But sex is a difficult subject to talk about—you know that. Sexual relationships are a very personal and private matter. And sex can be pretty complicated. The act itself is easy enough to describe (or is it? See chapters 3 and 4 for more on that), but all the identities, emotions, feelings, and sensations that go along with it are not. So, talking openly about personal, emotion-filled activities is not an easy thing to do for anyone. It takes practice, time, consideration, and thought.

What happens is that many young people end up with partial information about sex and sexual relationships. They collect bits and pieces from their classes, their families, what they see on television and in the movies, and what they are told in places of worship. Then, they try to fill in the rest of the information with what they hear from their friends, look up online, and learn from personal experiences. And that's how most of us learn about sex. It may not be totally accurate, but some information is better than none, right? Well, maybe. Some information is good, as long as that information is based in fact. Yet, our friends, television, and other media are not always accurate. It is difficult to figure out what is and is not true sometimes. That is where I hope to come in—to help you figure out what is and isn't accurate in the world of sex and relationships. Of course, some topics aren't always fact driven. Instead, topics like what are the most important aspects in a romantic relationship, the best way to keep yourself safer from STDs and unplanned pregnancy, and whether or not to come out require you to think about your own values and make your own decisions. Still, where I can, I try to provide you with the facts and contexts to help you be sexually safe, respectful, responsible, and happy.

Since There's Been Sex, There's Been Sexuality Education

Historians believe that the first sexuality education book, which was more of a sex manual, was written in China in 200 BC. The better-known ancient sexuality education manual, the *Kama Sutra*, was written in the third century AD. The original *Kama Sutra* had 1,000 chapters—more modern versions of the book have been edited to "only" 150 chapters. This book was quite progressive for its time, stating that it was important for both "youth" and women to be educated in sex, and that all responsible citizens appreciate the importance of sex education.[b]

What I Hope to Do in This Book

When it comes to sexuality education, I believe in using an approach called Rights, Respect, and Responsibility.[1] This means, I believe that:

- young people have the *right* to accurate information and quality health services;
- young people deserve *respect* when it comes to listening to their decisions about their sexual health and well-being
- society has a *responsibility* to provide young people with the tools they need to maintain their sexual health and have healthy, happy relationships

It was my intention to write a book that is inclusive and respectful of young people from different backgrounds. Hopefully, young people of different races, ethnicities, religious affiliations, sexual orientations, gender identities, and experiences find some things they can relate to as they read while also learning different perspectives. This brings me to some thoughts about gender identities and language. It was my goal to make the language in this book as gender inclusive as possible. However, because our society promotes a two-gender system (male, female), finding language to effectively communicate beyond this gender binary is challenging. Therefore, in some instances gender-specific words such as *boy* and *girl* are used in this book in order to communicate some concepts. This, however, does not mean that all people of a certain gender fit into the topics discussed, nor does it exclude people of different genders to whom the circumstances may apply. For example, not all people who menstruate are girls or women. I also understand that some people (including me) are not going to agree with the word choices used in some sections of this book. I hope in these cases you are able to read beyond the words used and see yourself in situations that you believe pertain to you.

Certainly, there is no way you are going to agree with everything I say, nor would I want you to. It's important to take the time to think about your own values when it comes to the best way to express your sexuality, form romantic relationships, and be sexually healthy. I provide medically accurate (and ideally practical) information and references, and include additional resources based on facts; hopefully these materials will help you when it comes to making your own sexual decisions—decisions that will be good for you and your partners. Yes, you'll already know some of the information in this book. I expect many of you will know a lot of the information I present here. But to tell the whole story, I need to repeat some information that you may already know. Besides, a little review never hurt anyone.

Sexuality is a complicated topic, so although this book is part of a series called "The Ultimate Teen Guide," no way can a sexuality education book be 100 percent complete. It is my goal to offer a brief overview of the essential stuff like healthy relationships and practicing safer sex, and also cover some topics that aren't as common in a sex education book such as how digital communications influence relationships and things to consider when dating someone older than or different from you. I hope that after you read this book you get some answers, but also start asking more questions about sexuality, your values, and how society portrays sexuality. In sum, I want to help you make your own decisions when it comes to having romantic relationships and being sexually healthy.

While often there is more than one answer to a particular question, I, as all humans do, have opinions. While I try to show different points of view throughout this book, to be honest I can't help myself and my biases are going to show

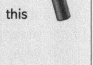

My Beliefs about Young People and Sexuality

When it comes to my beliefs about sexuality and sexuality education in young people, here are some of my basic beliefs that help shape this book. I believe that:

- young people have the right to ask questions about sex and get medically and scientifically accurate answers in return.
- young people already know a lot, but not all there is to know, about sex and relationships. Really, no one knows all there is to know and continual education is important.
- young people are going to make their own decisions about their sexuality and sexual health. Therefore, it's important for them to have access to information that can help them make the best decisions possible.
- getting information about a particular sexual topic doesn't mean anything about your sexual experiences or preferences. It just means you are curious.
- talking about sex is important in order to be sexually healthy and have healthy relationships.
- everyone has the right to feel comfortable and safe with their sexual decisions.

through. I do think that there is a "right" answer to some really difficult and controversial issues—but not all of them. My opinions and answers developed over time while doing research, teaching classes, and answering questions in magazines and on the Internet about teens, sex, and sexuality. They also developed as I gained experience in my own life. So, even though I believe this book can teach you a lot, I also think it's a good idea to get information from many places. Use the resources at the end of the book and talk to your family members and community to get different opinions. The more you learn, the more you know.

Who Is This Person, Anyway?

A fair question to ask is "Who is writing this book?" My name is L. Kris Gowen (the "L" stands for Laura, my first name, but I always go by Kris and Dr. Kris). I have a doctorate in adolescent development from Stanford University. This means that by the time I graduated from everything, I was technically in the twenty-first grade. It was a lot of work for sure, but overall I really liked being in school for all those years. There were times when I thought I wasn't going to make it, and I took time off from school and worked in between my different degrees (something I strongly suggest for any of you interested in graduate school), but overall I have no regrets being in school for that long.

While in graduate school, I did a lot of research on girls' body image as they go through puberty and on sexuality education. I wrote papers on how race and ethnicity relate to body image, how body image relates to dating, and how one's family styles influence romantic relationships among young people. I helped evaluate an AIDS prevention program that was taught by the local YWCA. I also began a stint of running online message boards and advice columns where teens can ask questions about sex and relationships. This has been my favorite thing to do. You will see some of the questions I received, along with my answers, in this book.

After school, I continued to be an online sexpert and taught human sexuality courses to university and graduate students. I also taught teachers how to teach sex education (say that ten times fast), and how to reach out to any of their students they felt needed a bit of support. A word about all those teachers—you may not believe it, but they care an awful lot about you. They worry and want to help. If ever you feel that you need an adult to talk to, and your parents are not an option, think about talking to a teacher.

When I am not dealing with anything related to sex education, I am either hanging out with my friends or traveling—I've been to South Korea, Vietnam, and the Middle East, as well as several other countries. I also love hockey and karaoke.

Thanks for taking the time to read the introduction. I hope that it gives you a basic idea as to who I am and where this book may take you. In short, what I hope to do is provide you with honest answers to honest questions about sex and relationships. If you read this book and come away with new knowledge or just end up feeling more comfortable about making sexual decisions, then I've done my job.

Happy reading!

BODY BASICS

In this chapter, basic sexual and reproductive anatomy are discussed, as well as fertility and sexual pleasure. Our world typically divides people into two neat categories—male and female—and as a result some of the language used in this chapter reflects this approach to simplify some concepts. However, sex and gender are not simple concepts—far from it. Both are spectrums, meaning that there are more than two sexes (male and female) and more than two genders (girl/woman and boy/man; see chapter 2 for more on this). This means that not all people who identify as a certain sex or gender will be able to generalize what is happening to their bodies with what is outlined in the text. I support those of you who do not agree or fit in with the word choices used here (I don't agree with all of them either), and understand that some readers aren't going to relate to certain sections that attempt to describe their sex or gender; that's OK. It was not my intention to exclude anyone, and I hope people are able to use the information in this chapter to help better understand and love their bodies.

Reviewing Puberty

Puberty is the time when bodies develop and change in order to become fertile. This means that, at the end of puberty, a body is ready to be involved in making a baby—but the person who inhabits that body might not be! For young people, puberty begins anywhere between the ages of eight and sixteen years (though sometimes earlier and sometimes later than that), and lasts about two or three years. During this time, bodies of all types go through many changes, including changes in hormones, voice, height, and weight. Hair will grow in armpits and in the genital area. In some people, the first sign of puberty is the beginning of breast development. Body odor may become a problem as armpit sweat glands become active (deodorant and bathing can help with that).

Another common occurrence during puberty is the "wet dream," which is simply having an orgasm, or experiencing wetness from sexual arousal, while sleeping. People of all genders have wet dreams, but it is more noticeable if you have a penis because the emissions happen outside the body as opposed to inside the vagina. However, not all people have wet dreams—it is normal to have or not have them while going through puberty, or even as you go through life.

Males and females also experience different changes. During midpuberty, young people go through a "growth spurt," during which they get both taller and heavier. Sometimes a person can grow four inches taller in just one year! Guys will gain more muscle, while girls will gain more fat. It is common for some girls to gain twenty-four pounds of fat during the two or three years of puberty.[1] In fact, during puberty, a girl's body fat content can rise from about 8 percent to about 25 percent. This increase in the amount of fat on the body is needed to help it get ready for pregnancy and carrying a baby to term.

Fertility

Different bodies change in different ways to prepare for fertility. While not everyone will be able to have children later in life (and not everyone will choose to, either), here are the basics of fertility.

Getting to Know Yourself and Your Body

Some of you can see your genitals more easily than others. However, everyone should take time to get to know their bodies and check out what their genitals look like. If you don't, you can have a hard time understanding your reproductive anatomy. You also may have a more difficult time understanding your sexual responses without investigating those parts of your body. There is nothing shameful about taking a look "down there" to see what it's all about. To see a vulva, clitoris, and vagina, sit with your legs apart and use a mirror. You might have to separate the labia (lips) to see the whole picture, but it's well worth it. Depending on your angle, you may even be able to see your cervix. (If you can't and are curious to know what a cervix looks like, check out the photo gallery at beautifulcervix.com.) It might be easier to see a penis, but it's still important to take a close look at all its parts and also look at the scrotum. By becoming familiar with what your body looks and feels like when it's healthy, you are better able to realize if something doesn't look right, and be able to tell your doctor about it. You can also better communicate with your partner about where you do and don't like to be touched.

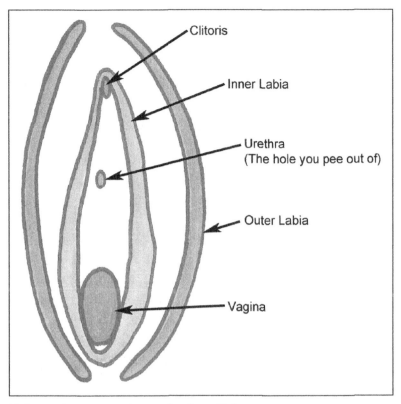

Vulva and company. *Image by Amy Nelson*

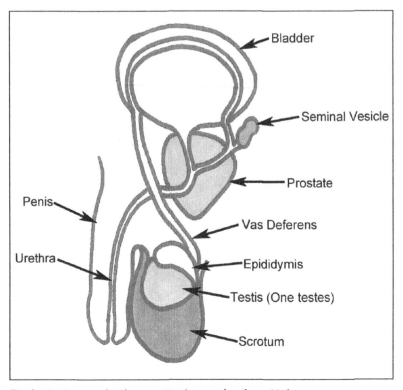

Penis, testes, and other parts. *Image by Amy Nelson*

Getting Pregnant

There is only one way for a pregnancy to happen—a sperm has to fertilize an egg. Due to the wonders of science, this phenomenon can happen outside of the human body. However, for this book we are only concerned about pregnancies that happen during vaginal intercourse. Women can only get pregnant during certain times of the month, called ovulation. As explained later, ovulation occurs once per fertility cycle, when the ovaries release an egg. If sperm happens to be around a female when the egg is released (or are still alive inside the uterus or fallopian tube when the egg is released), there is a good chance that a pregnancy will happen.

Many people believe that as long as vaginal intercourse happens outside of ovulation, then there is no chance of pregnancy. While this is true in theory, there are many problems with this line of thinking. First of all, it's very difficult to predict when ovulation will occur—it can even happen during menstruation (so, no, having sex during one's period is not a good form of birth control!). This is especially true for young people whose periods have not been occurring long enough to establish a regular pattern. Remember that stress, diet, travel, and other things can all prevent a menstrual cycle from being regular. Now think about the average teen whose periods have only been around for a few years, who also may be expe-

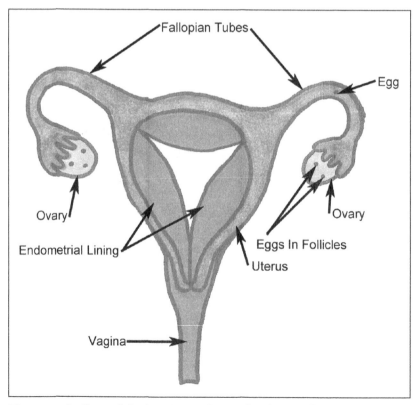

Uterus and other related anatomy. *Image by Amy Nelson*

riencing a lot of stress and may not be eating the healthiest. Predicting a young person's menstrual cycle becomes almost impossible, and thus knowing when a pregnancy can and cannot happen is an equally challenging task. Then you also need to consider the lifetime of the sperm. Sperm can stay alive in the vagina and uterus for up to six days. So, even if you know when ovulation will happen, you don't know how long the sperm will live inside the female's body. This makes trying to figure out what days are "safe" to have sex even more difficult. There are classes where couples can learn how to predict when having sex will lead to pregnancy, and when it will not. It takes one to two years to go through these classes, which are run by a trained professional.

If it takes at least one year of careful instruction to learn how to predict ovulation, trying to figure out how to do it on your own doesn't sound like such a good idea. There are many different birth control methods and sex alternatives available to you, and using one of those is a much better idea than trying to guess when it is and is not safe to have sex in order to avoid pregnancy. That said, it's still important to know what happens during fertility cycles, so read on!

Menstrual Cycle: How It Really Works

Your period, your "time of the month," your "Aunt Flo"— whatever you call it, most girls experience it for the first time between the ages of nine and sixteen, and every month (twenty-eight days or so) after that. A first period doesn't usually happen until one or two years after the first signs of puberty. First, the vagina, ovaries, and uterus grow, and many girls get a clear or white discharge from their vagina. Then menses, or a first period, will happen. The clitoris grows larger as do the vaginal "lips," or labia. Pubic hair also gets coarser and grows a lot more. During this time, the young woman continues to grow a bit taller and larger, and breasts finish developing.

The funny thing is, although most people know it happens, the purpose of menstruation and how it works remain a mystery to many. This is a sad thing. Knowing how the human body works allows us to appreciate it that much more. Knowing how and why women menstruate allows people to unlock the mystery of the fertility cycle.

The bottom-line purpose of menstruation is so that a woman can get pregnant. Each month, an egg is released by one of two ovaries. The egg travels to the uterus by way of the fallopian tubes. The idea here is that once the egg is released, it will be fertilized by sperm and be on its way to becoming a fetus and then a baby.

Next, in order for the egg/future baby to be comfortable, the uterus starts to develop a thick, cushy lining made up of blood and nutrients, while the egg is making its way down the fallopian tube. In a way, the uterus is getting ready for its "house guest"—one that it thinks will stay for about nine months. Most of the time, however, the egg is not fertilized and disintegrates inside the body. Since the uterus has no one staying in it, it doesn't need all that nutrient-rich lining it created. So, it sheds this lining through the vagina. It is this lining that is the blood of a period. This cycle of egg release and uterus preparation will happen once every three to six weeks or so until the ovaries stop releasing eggs. The menstrual cycle and the associated periods go on for about thirty years, sometimes more.

However, this description of the menstrual cycle is missing something important—the hormones! In fact, many people associate menstruation with hormones being totally out of whack. This is not the case. While it's true that hormone levels change with the menstrual cycle, they do so for very distinct reasons. These reasons are divided into three phases described next. In these descriptions, the days given for when the phases start are based on a twenty-eight-day cycle. Since cycles can be shorter or longer, these are only estimates.

The Menstrual Phase
(day zero to day five, give or take)

The menstrual phase is basically the time you have your period. During this time, the endometrium (that cushy nutrient-filled lining built by the uterus) is shed, along with a little blood. Meanwhile, the body gets ready for the next egg to come along. Small pulses of gonadotropin-releasing hormone from the hypothalamus (a part of your brain) lead to small pulses of *luteinizing* hormone (LH) and follicle stimulating hormone (FSH) from the pituitary gland. LH and FSH stimulate several follicles (each containing an egg cell) to develop in the ovaries. Usually only the strongest egg will survive this process and enter into the next phase (when more eggs mature in a cycle, it's possible for twins, triplets, or more).

The Follicular/Proliferative Phase
(about days six to fourteen)

Now, only the strongest egg or eggs have matured enough for eventual release—this egg (or these eggs, in some cases) is the survivor of this menstrual round and will continue through the process, while the rest of the eggs wait for another time. The FSH continues promoting the growth of this chosen egg and also tells the body that it's time to increase the level of estrogen. This rise in estrogen acts as a signal for the uterus to start making its lining. The follicle (egg) continues to grow, getting itself ready for fertilization after release. When the level of estrogen peaks, that's the signal for the egg that the time is right, and off it goes on its journey toward possible fertilization.

Ovulation! The Time of Fertility
(midcycle, but a woman is at risk for a pregnancy for more days than just a couple out of every month)

Estrogen is at its max point, and the follicle cage releases the egg. This process is known as ovulation. The ovum (one egg) then travels from the ovary down the fallopian tube and into the uterus. Now that the egg is released, the level of estrogen goes down, but not too much, as it still has to help build that lining in the uterus.

The Luteal/Secretory Phase
(days sixteen to twenty-eight or so)

Once the ovum is released, the follicle it broke out of becomes a sac known as the corpus luteum. LH causes the corpus luteum to grow and to secrete progesterone, yet another hormone needed for pregnancy. The progesterone makes the endometrial lining stronger, so that the uterus is ready for a baby. When pregnancy doesn't happen during ovulation, the level of progesterone peaks about a week after ovulation and then begins to drop along with the estrogen level. The flow of blood to the lining decreases, and at that point the lining breaks and sheds during

Dealing with Periods throughout History

There have been products to help control menstrual flow for almost all of history. The first references to tampons have been found in hieroglyphics—the writing of ancient Egypt—as early as 1550 BC! The first commercial tampons in the United States weren't sold until the early 1930s, however. Before tampons, cloth napkins were used to absorb blood. Although disposable pads were available in Europe as early as the 1890s, it was not until the 1920s that they were available in the United States.[a]

menstruation. The dip in estrogen and progesterone at the end of the cycle helps let the body know that it's time to start the cycle all over again.

That's how hormones get the body ready to have a baby and deal with the fact that no baby is coming, should the egg not be fertilized. If an egg were to be fertilized during this time, that is, if pregnancy did occur, the levels of estrogen and progesterone would stay high in order for the lining in the uterus to stay healthy and fresh. Because these hormone levels would not decrease, the menstrual cycle would not be signaled to start again. This is why pregnant women don't get their periods. There is no lining to shed—it's being used to feed the fetus inside.

Irregular Periods

Now that we spent all that time talking about the menstrual cycle, it is important to know that a menstrual cycle is more often irregular than regular. In other words, it is a lot more common for a period to happen at unexpected times than at expected times. This is especially true when periods first begin. As a teen gets older, periods often become more predictable. Things like stress, diet, not getting enough sleep, and a crazy schedule can all make a period start and stop at strange times. Read these questions and answers to learn more.

Question:
I started my period about two years ago and I still do not have it regularly. I skip several months before having one. It had been a long time (five to six) months since my last one. I don't feel comfortable talking to my mom and I don't have a regular doctor. Is this normal? What should I do? Is there a pill/vitamin I can take to have a period every month?
—Age seventeen

Answer:
You don't mention if you are sexually active or not. If you are sexually active and haven't had your period for five or six months, you need to check a pregnancy test right away. If you haven't been sexually active, it is not that uncommon to still have irregular periods at your age. One option for dealing with irregular periods is to start on birth control pills. In this case, the pill is not used for birth control (unless you are also sexually active), but for regulating the timing of your period. You should make an appointment with a primary care provider (a family practitioner or general internist) or with an obstetrician/gynecologist for a checkup and to discuss your concerns.
Signed,
Dr. X, We Are Talking, teen health website

Question:

I just got spotting today, and thought my period is starting, but all afternoon it's just been spotting! I don't know if it's staying or leaving??? Also, my cycle has changed! I usually get my periods at the end of the month, but today is April 4!! I'm not sexually active, so I know I'm not pregnant.

What is this?? I'm confused??? Please answer back. Thanks.[2]

—Age eighteen

Answer:

It is very common for young people to have intermenstrual spotting and occasional change in their menstrual cycle from normal. This can happen in relation to emotional stress or depression, increased exercise, fasting or dieting, and sometimes from a missed ovulation cycle (i.e., ovulation does not take place) and so the hormonal cycle gets disrupted. You should not worry, this sometimes resolves after one or two cycles. If, however, you start having persistent intermenstrual spotting or a persistent irregularity in your menstrual cycle then you should come in for an evaluation.

Signed,

Dr. X, We Are Talking, teen health website

Sports and Periods

You may have heard (or experienced) that many girls do not get their periods when they are seriously involved in athletics. Almost any female who is in serious training for any sport is at risk for developing secondary amenorrhea, which is the medical term for the stopping of the monthly period after it has been happening for a while. Many things can cause secondary amenorrhea in athletes—stress, a

For More Information on Menstruation

There is a whole website dedicated to the history of menstruation, www .mum.org. Check out what women used as tampons throughout history, read about religion and menstruation, or learn about getting your period from a Kotex instruction booklet from 1938! Even get some great jokes about that "little friend." It is all here.

low percentage of body fat, and rapid weight loss are some of the culprits. Overall, the more active and vigorous the sport, the more likely there will be irregular, if not absent, periods. Scientists and doctors have mixed opinions as to whether experiencing secondary amenorrhea is dangerous—some think that not getting a period for a while puts a young person at risk for osteoporosis (a bone-thinning disease).[3] For now, it's recommended that if you do not get your period for three months in a row, talk to a doctor about it to look for possible causes and solutions. Also, it's not clear whether girls who don't get their periods for a long time will get them again on their own once athletic training is less intense.

PMS

The changes in hormones that are responsible for menstruation can also cause emotional and physical changes during a cycle. The medical term for these changes is *premenstrual syndrome*, or PMS. PMS was first recognized as a medical condition in 1931, but historical descriptions of the emotional and physical changes that go along with a menstrual cycle have been discovered to reach as far back as Hippocrates's writings from the fifth century BC.[4]

About 85 percent of menstruating women in the United States experience some form of PMS, although the symptoms and their intensity vary tremendously from person to person. Some get very moody in an angry way, others in a sad way. Some get very tender breasts, others get super-awful cramps. No two women have the same type of PMS. Researchers believe that 20 to 40 percent of women who have PMS experience symptoms that make life difficult; another 2 to 5 percent report that their PMS is challenging enough that it takes over their lives.[5]

No one is exactly sure what causes PMS, but medical experts believe it's caused by a combination of things—physiological, genetic, nutritional, and behavioral reasons are likely to all be involved. Some even think a change in attitude about menstruation can make PMS symptoms less severe. There are, however, many ways to help someone feel better when they have PMS. Exercising can really help, as can other forms of stress reduction. Eating less refined sugar and cutting out caffeine and alcohol can also help reduce the symptoms of PMS. Finally, over-the-counter drugs such as ibuprofen are also effective.

Discharge: A Normal Part of Having a Vagina

The word *discharge* often conjures up images of sexually transmitted diseases. Discharge is seen as unhealthy and unwanted. But, in reality, all vaginas have discharge; discharge is simply fluids from the vagina that leave the body. An answer to a question about discharge by someone from the We Are Talking teen health website talks about all the different types of discharge and what they might mean.

Question:

What causes brown discharge? I haven't gotten my period in a while but recently I got a brown discharge. It only happened one day and hasn't since.

—Age sixteen

Answer:

Vaginal discharge is normal and varies during your menstrual cycle. Before ovulation (the release of the egg), there is a lot of mucous produced, up to thirty times more than after ovulation. It is also more watery and elastic during that phase of your cycle. You may want to wear panty liners during that time. Discharge is abnormal only if it has a yellow or green color, is clumpy like cottage cheese, or has a bad odor. If you are worried, see a doctor.

Here are some descriptions of different types of discharge:

- *White:* Thick, white discharge is common at the beginning and end of your cycle. White discharge that looks like cottage cheese and is itchy often indicates a yeast infection. This can be treated by over-the-counter creams or suppositories.
- *Clear and stretchy:* This is "fertile" mucous and means you are ovulating, or will ovulate soon.
- *Clear and watery:* This occurs at different times of your cycle and can be particularly heavy after exercising.
- *Yellow or green:* This may indicate an infection, especially in a large amount or if it has a foul odor.
- *Brown:* This may happen right after periods and is just "cleaning out" your vagina. Old blood looks brown.
- *Spotting blood/brown:* This may occur when you are ovulating/during midcycle. But if your period is late or scanty, pregnancy is possible. Check a first-morning urine sample for pregnancy.

Maturing Testes and Sperm

Unlike eggs, which exist as soon as a person is born, sperm are not produced until testes go through puberty and mature. The first sign of this process is when the testes (balls) start to grow, and the scrotum (the wrinkled skin that holds the testes) turns darker. By midpuberty pubic hair can be seen, and the penis starts to get larger. During this time, sperm begin to be produced. As the testes begin to make sperm and other parts of the body create the ejaculatory fluid ("cum"), semen is produced for the first time. In fact, semen production is highest in the early stages of puberty because hormone levels are highest during this time of life (this is also the reason so many erections happen during this time). Once this process begins, the testes will continue to make mature sperm that are capable of fertilizing an egg (health issues that may impact fertility aside).

Sperm and Semen

Sperm, half of the equation to baby making (ova being the other half), are made in the testes (also known as "balls"). The testes hang away from the body because in order for the sperm to develop properly, they must stay at a slightly lower temperature (95° to 97° Fahrenheit, 35° to 36° Celsius) than normal body temperature (98.6° F, 37° C).

Once the sperm are made, they have to travel from each testis to a coiled tube on the outer surface of each testis called the epididymis, where they mature in around three weeks. Sperm exit the body through the penis during ejaculation. When the penis is stimulated, it becomes erect, and ejaculation propels mature sperm from the epididymis through a long tube (vas deferens or ductus deferens) inside the body. While the sperm is traveling through the body, it gets mixed with nutrient-rich fluids from the seminal vesicles and a milky secretion from the prostate gland. The sperm and fluids together are known as semen or cum.

Semen does three things:

1. Provides a watery environment in which the sperm cells can swim while outside the body
2. Provides nutrients for the sperm cells
3. Protects the sperm cells by neutralizing acids in the vagina and fallopian tubes

Thanks to all the fluids in the semen, the sperm can leave the penis in a protected environment full of nutrients and acid-fighting materials so that it has a better chance of surviving and making its way through the vagina, then the cervix, then the uterus, then the fallopian tubes to fertilize an egg.

Pre-ejaculate

Pre-ejaculate (also known as pre-cum) is that little bit of lubricant that you may notice at the tip of an erect penis before ejaculation happens. This fluid helps protect the sperm against the acids in the urethra (caused by urine) and also gives the sperm an extra slippery boost upon ejaculation. It's important to know that pre-ejaculate can have sperm in it, as well as any STD (sexually transmitted disease) bacteria or virus. Therefore, it's not a good idea to let an erect penis get near another person's openings, where that individual might get an STD or become pregnant.

Predicting Fertility

There is only one way for a pregnancy to happen—a sperm has to fertilize an egg. Due to the wonders of science, this can happen outside as well as inside the human body. However, for this book we are only focusing on pregnancies that happen during vaginal intercourse.

Pregnancy can only happen during certain times of the month, during ovulation. Ovulation occurs once every three to six weeks, sometimes more, sometimes less. When ovaries release an egg and sperm happen to be around, pregnancy can occur. Many people believe that as long as two people have vaginal intercourse while ovulation is not occurring, there is no chance of pregnancy. There are some flaws in this thinking. First of all, it's difficult to predict ovulation—ovulation can even happen during menstruation! This is especially true for young women, whose periods have not been around long enough to settle into a regular pattern (note: periods can be regular, then irregular, and then regular again throughout life). Remember—stress, diet, travel, and other things can all prevent a menstrual cycle from being regular. Now think about the average young female, whose periods have only been around for a few years. There's often a lot of stress and diet changes happening, making predicting a menstrual cycle challenging. Therefore, predicting when fertilization can and cannot happen is equally challenging.

It's also important to consider the lifespan of sperm. Sperm can stay alive in the vagina, uterus, and fallopian tubes for up to six days. So, even if you know when ovulation will occur, you can't really tell how long sperm will be around to fertilize the egg. This makes it difficult to figure out what days are "safe" to have vaginal intercourse if you don't want pregnancy.

Pregnancy

If you think you could be pregnant, it's important to find out sooner rather than later. The earlier you find out, the more options you have. First of all, finding out there *isn't* an unplanned pregnancy can reduce stress and give you a chance to figure out if you need to reassess your birth control options (see chapter 6 for many options). Finding out about a pregnancy in the early stages allows you the option of early prenatal (before birth) care or abortion (see chapter 12). The first three months are an important time for the fetus, and getting good prenatal care is essential during this time. So do yourself and the fetus a favor—get a pregnancy test as soon as you start to feel any signs!

There are a few early signs of pregnancy. Not everyone who is pregnant will feel all of them or even some of them. The most obvious is missing a period. If you miss a period, don't jump to conclusions: missing a period is common and doesn't always indicate pregnancy. But, if you do miss a period, look for these other signs of early pregnancy:

- Nausea/vomiting/feeling queasy—sometimes referred to as "morning sickness," but it can happen any time of the day
- Soreness or enlargement of the breasts
- Increased need to urinate because the fetus is pushing on the bladder
- Feeling faint or tired
- Just "feeling pregnant"—exhausted, hungry, achy, different from how you were before

There are two ways you can get a pregnancy test: at a clinic or by taking a home pregnancy test. There are many good reasons for each. A home test is more private. If you get tested at a clinic, you can make sure it's more accurate and you will be in a place where you can discuss options with a professional based on the result. Studies show that some pregnancy tests can be very confusing so that results are read correctly less than half the time. In other words, people are more likely to read results of home tests incorrectly than correctly—another reason getting tested at a clinic might be the best way to go.

Pregnancy tests work by measuring a hormone the body starts producing after the fertilized egg begins to grow. For that reason, it's important to wait at least two weeks after vaginal intercourse to get an accurate test result. Waiting these two weeks gives your body a chance to create enough hormone to cause the test to turn positive if there is a pregnancy. If you take the test too early, there's a chance of getting a result that says you aren't pregnant when you are.

Whether done at the clinic or at home, a pregnancy test works by measuring the amount of this hormone in your urine (pee). It's best to take a urine sample from your first bathroom trip of the morning. This is because early morning urine is more concentrated since you haven't gone to the bathroom in a while. The more concentrated the urine, the more likely you'll get an accurate test.

The Challenges of Pregnancy

Whether or not birth control is used, if vaginal intercourse takes place, there's a chance that pregnancy can occur. Obviously, the more effective the birth control used, the less chance of pregnancy. But things happen. If you find yourself involved in an unplanned pregnancy, there are a few options. Abortion and adoption are discussed in chapter 12. You can also carry the pregnancy to term and become a parent.

Having a baby when you are young can be challenging. Biologically, young women who give birth are at greater risk for developing complications. Also, the fetus is more likely to be born prematurely and/or have low birth weight. Finishing your education becomes more difficult, too. Fewer than half of teen mothers finish high school, and only 2 percent graduate from college by the time they are thirty; teen fathers also have a decreased chance of finishing high school and going on for more schooling.[6] A lower level of education seriously limits job opportunities down the line, so young parents are also less likely to find jobs that pay well. Parenting costs a lot of money with the additional expenses of food, clothes, toys, equipment (car seats, strollers, etc.), and child care. Socially, it will be harder for young parents to hang out with their friends, engage in hobbies, and spend some good alone time with themselves or their partner. Having a child probably means you will need to put some of your dreams on hold, but you will be able to pick those up later. Don't lose sight of them! As a parent, you will need to learn a bunch of new skills—everything from changing a diaper to helping your baby go to sleep. Good news is, there are many websites that can help you sort through the changes in your life. Start with www.sexetc.org and look around their "Pregnancy" section for stories, advice, and resources. There may be new parent support groups in your community that could be helpful. There is also a book in this series by Jessica Akin called *Pregnancy and Parenting: The Ultimate Teen Guide*[7] that provides excellent information for pregnant and parenting young people.

While having a family when you are young is challenging, with the right support and strategy you can raise a child successfully. Plenty of children's clothing and supplies are available at thrift stores and by asking other people with young children for hand-me-downs. There are often support groups and communities for young parents—search online or ask your local social services department for ideas. You can also meet other parents by going to a playground or community center and share your experiences. Parenting is a very emotional experience—the highs and lows will all be felt. Finding someone to talk to that you trust—another parent (maybe your own), a counselor, religious leader, or other adult—can really help. Get advice from people you admire who are already parents. No matter how it feels sometimes, you are not alone.

Teen Pregnancy: Know the Facts

Here are some basic facts about teen pregnancy in the United States:

1. Each year, more than six hundred thousand young women aged fifteen to nineteen become pregnant.
2. Over 80 percent of pregnancies in girls aged fifteen to nineteen are unplanned. These unplanned teen pregnancies make up about one-fifth of all unintended pregnancies each year.
3. More than half (60 percent) of teen pregnancies end in birth, while about one in four end in abortion; the rest end in a miscarriage.
4. The three states that have the highest rates of young parents are New Mexico, Mississippi, and Texas.[b]

Know Your Rights

Some pregnant youth or young parents face discrimination regarding education, employment, custody, and other issues. If you think you are being treated unfairly or illegally because of your status as a parent or parent-to-be, find out more about your rights at aclu.org/pregnant-and-parenting-teens.

About Penises

Teen boys seem to worry about penises a lot. And this concern does not always go away with age; grown men also can spend much too much time worrying about something they can do nothing about. While it is true that not all penises are the same size, they are generally between three and a half to four and a half inches when soft and five to seven inches when erect. A smaller penis will increase in size more than a larger penis when it becomes erect, so those concerned about a smaller soft penis might take comfort in knowing that when erect, a smaller penis can make up ground.

Please be assured that size does not matter when it comes to how many orgasms one can have, how fertile someone is, or how well a person can satisfy a partner sexually. Communication, a good relationship, and true care for your partner make for a good sexual relationship. The size of your penis will not matter if you truly care about your partner and are interested in having a healthy sexual relationship.

Circumcision

Circumcision, the surgical removal of the foreskin on the penis, is one of the oldest surgeries in history, having been performed for thousands of years. On an uncircumcised penis, the foreskin covers the glans, or the tip, of the penis. On a circumcised penis, the glans is exposed. Circumcision sometimes is performed on infants for religious reasons; people who practice Judaism or Islam are more likely to believe a penis should be circumcised. Circumcision for nonreligious reasons is also common in different cultures, for example, in sub-Saharan Africa and in many ethnic groups around the world, such as aboriginal Australians, the Aztecs and Mayan, and inhabitants of the Philippines, eastern Indonesia, and various Pacific Islands, including Fiji and the Polynesian islands. Among these cultures, circumcision is seen as a rite of passage into adulthood, and thus it is performed on older boys.[8]

Circumcision can also be done for health reasons. Some believe that it's better to remove the foreskin in order to avoid infections; however, as long as an uncircumcised penis is washed along with the area underneath the foreskin, infections should not be a problem. Circumcision does *not* decrease the risk of penile cancer as once thought, but it may decrease the likelihood of contracting HIV. About 70 percent of penises are circumcised in the United States at birth; in contrast, only about 30 percent of penises are circumcised worldwide.[9]

Questions about Penises

People have a lot of questions when it comes to penises. Here are some to help you think about what is normal and perhaps not-so-normal when it comes to this part of the body. If you at any time believe that something might be wrong with you, do yourself a favor and ask a doctor about it. It is better to be safe than sorry!

Question:
    Why do some people have penises that look different? Some have skin that cover the head of their penis and others do not. Is there a health

reason for this or is it because some just want to be different? I saw one with a bunch of skin and it was strange looking.

—Curious

Answer:

Great question! A penis with skin on it has not been circumcised. Many parents choose to circumcise their baby's penis—this means that they remove the skin that covers the head of the penis (this skin is called the foreskin). If a baby is not circumcised, then there will be extra skin on a penis, like the one you saw.

People circumcise their babies for religious reasons and for health reasons. Some people think that being circumcised makes it easier to keep the penis clean and prevents it from getting infected. But as long as the person washes the penis and makes sure the spot under the foreskin is cleaned, all is okay.

—Dr. Kris

Question:

I know that a bent penis is very common but my problem is that it seems to be crooked. When I get an erection it isn't straight but rather points more to one side—not that it is perpendicular to my leg but still. I don't think it has always been like this but I'm not positive. Is this normal? I'm not having sex right now but will it complicate sexual intercourse? Could masturbation be the cause of this? Is there any way to straighten it out?

—Seventeen-year-old

Answer:

Penis sizes vary considerably and many have a penis that bends to one side or another or "stands straight up" when erect. It will not matter at all—sex is about relationships and intimacy—pleasing a partner includes many things not related to penis size (or crookedness)—and the quality of the interaction can be measured by how well you learn what makes your partner feel good, emotionally and physically.

Try not to worry,

Dr. X, We Are Talking, teen health website

Question:

I was wondering does the amount of testosterone in your body affect penis growth? I have heard that more testosterone in the body shrinks the penis. Is that true?

—Seventeen-year-old

Answer:

Testosterone is necessary to cause the penis to develop and to grow normally. Having too much testosterone is very rare, but it does not cause any problems with growth and development of the penis.

Good Luck,

Dr. X, We Are Talking, teen health website

Question:

I am uncircumcised and it hurts to touch the head of my penis sometimes. Could there be something wrong?

—Eighteen-year-old

Answer:

The head of the penis is sensitive in everybody. Masturbating can certainly cause it to be sensitive, especially if it is done without any lubricant (such as a water soluble lubricant like KY jelly). As long as the foreskin can be pulled back to allow the head of the penis to be cleaned, the foreskin is not a problem. It is important to pull the foreskin back down, covering the head of the penis after it is cleaned.

Good Luck,

Dr. X, We Are Talking, teen health website[10]

Testicular Cancer

Cancer of the testicles accounts for only about 1 percent of all cancers in men, *but* it is the most common type of cancer in males aged fifteen to thirty-five. The good news is that testicular cancer is almost always curable if it's found early. Therefore, if you have any lumps or swelling in your testes, it doesn't necessarily mean you have cancer, but you should be checked by your health-care provider. Here are some other symptoms that may hint that you might have testicular cancer:

- A lump in either testicle, ranging in size from a pea to a golf ball
- Any enlargement or swelling of a testicle
- A significant shrinking of a testicle
- A change in the hardness of a testicle
- A feeling of heaviness in the scrotum
- A dull ache in the lower abdomen or in the groin
- A sudden collection of fluid in the scrotum
- Pain or discomfort in a testicle or in the scrotum

If you have some of these symptoms, talk to your doctor as soon as possible.

The Hymen

The vagina is partially covered by a thin membrane (like a piece of skin) called the hymen. The hymen is also known as the "cherry" in slang terms. The hymen usually does not cover the entire vaginal opening, since there must be some way for the menstrual fluid, or period, to leave the body. This membrane, although it has very little biological purpose, has great cultural significance. Some believe that the existence of an intact hymen on a woman means that she is still a virgin (and some women who talk about having sex for the first time talk about having their "cherry popped"). However, many women who have not had sex yet have their hymens separated, torn, or stretched through exercise or using a tampon. Sometimes the hymen separates for no clear reason. Those who do not have their hymens torn prior to having sex for the first time may feel some pain and notice some bleeding the first time they have sex.

Question:

I was just wondering where that layer of skin, the hymen, is exactly. Is it right when you enter the vagina, or further in?

—Curious eighteen-year-old in Kentucky

Answer:

It is farther in, approximately one inch.

Sincerely,

Dr. X, We Are Talking, teen health website

Question:

My boyfriend and I have been dating for five and a half years and recently we decided to start having sex. Once during sex, my hymen broke all the way, so it is no longer a ring but now just two small separate pieces. Although they are not painful, they are uncomfortable because they kind of just "hang out" of my vagina. Is this normal and is there anything I can do about them?

—An eighteen-year-old in Virginia

Answer:

This does sound like a normal occurrence after the hymen breaks. In some, the remaining pieces of the broken hymen hang down, and in others they are not noticeable. After a few months this tissue will likely shrink and not bother you anymore. If it does bother you after a few months, you can have it removed, usually by a gynecologist.

Sincerely,

Dr. X, We Are Talking, teen health website

Question:

Ever since I started my period I could never get a tampon in. It wouldn't go in at all, and I wasn't nervous. I tried every way possible. When my boyfriend fingered me his finger couldn't even get halfway in, it's like there's something blocking there. Then after a while of trying I get this terrible, hot, burning feeling in my vaginal area. It's a terrible pain. I then tried to get a tampon in after he fingered me and it went almost halfway in, and it didn't hurt, but there was no way to get it any further in there.

What's wrong with me? I'm very afraid; this has been going on for years now.

—Age seventeen

Answer:

There is probably nothing wrong. If you haven't had sexual intercourse then your vaginal opening may be too small to accommodate a tampon. Digital manipulation (fingering) through sexual foreplay can stretch the hymen, the thin skin layer that partly covered the vaginal opening. Also have your doctor examine you to see if the hymen is fairly tight and needs some stretching, or even a small snip to widen it to accommodate a tampon. You can also go to your doctor and ask her to help you insert a tampon. Do not be embarrassed, she can help.

Hang in there,

Dr. X, We Are Talking, teen health website

Breasts

Every body has breasts; it's just that in some bodies, the breasts grow more than in others. Breasts are relatively simple parts of the body, made up of connective tissue and fat. In women, breasts also have milk (mammary) glands and ducts. Breasts start growing around age eight or nine and finish growing by age seventeen or eighteen (though breasts can get bigger and smaller as people gain and lose weight). Breasts do not have any muscles; no matter what exercises a person performs, breasts will not get any bigger. Creams, pills, and other products don't work either. The only way to increase the size of a breast is to gain weight; more fat means more breast.

Many women, unfortunately, complain about their breasts. They feel their breasts are too big, too small, or too lopsided. They believe their nipples are too brown, too small, or too pointy. The truth is, there are as many types of breasts as there are people; no two pairs of breasts are alike, and for that matter, no two breasts are alike. What I mean is that no one has completely symmetrical breasts, especially young people; for some reason, the two breasts will sometimes grow at different rates, and thus a person will look lopsided until their breasts are done growing. Even after full maturity, however, all natural breasts are lopsided and many breasts will be different enough in size that it's noticeable if you stare (but really, people tend to not look that closely without being intimate—that's rude!). Same thing goes for nipples. Nipples come in all different sizes and shapes, and no one has the same nipples as anyone else.

Why does our society care about breasts so much? Really, all they're there for is to be a source of food for an infant after a woman gives birth. But as you all know, the significance of breasts as a sexual part of females gives them a whole new status among body parts. They are stared at, gawked at, and sometimes touched. Breasts, especially the nipples, can actually be a very sensitive and erotic place on a body—nipples will often get hard and erect from any sort of stimulation, such as touch and cold weather. This is because the nipple is made of erectile tissue, just like a penis or a clitoris. But not all people like to have their breasts or nipples touched during intimate moments. And *no one* should have their breasts touched by random people who for whatever reason think they have the right to do it. Breasts are unique in that they are a sexual body part that can be seen through clothing. But just because anyone can see them does not mean that anyone can touch them.

Orgasms and Sexual Response

People sometimes experience orgasms at the peak of their sexual arousal and excitement. Orgasms consist of a tensing and releasing of muscles in a series of contractions. Sometimes these muscle contractions happen all throughout the body, while sometimes the muscle contractions are more focused in the genital and/or groin area. It's really hard to describe what an orgasm feels like, as it feels different to different people, and it can even feel different to the same person in different situations. Some people feel orgasms as a huge rush, while others feel more of a tickle, and then a sense of relief. Some people feel them all over their body, while others feel them just around the genital area. Sometimes parts of the body go numb or feel like they are asleep, while at other times the whole body may feel a big "whoosh" as it reaches climax. Some people make noise, some laugh, some stay quiet. Sexual expression is very different from person to person, and there is no right or wrong way to react. When random people are asked to write down what an orgasm feels like to them, it's hard for other people to tell what gender they are, who their partner was, or what body parts were involved; in other words, the plumbing among people may be different, but the feelings people have during orgasm are both unique and similar.

Orgasms are often reached through the stimulation of a penis or clitoris. The clitoris is a small, sensitive organ whose sole purpose is to provide sexual pleasure. It's located right above the vagina and can look like a small button or knob. The clitoris often "hides" underneath a fold of skin called the clitoral hood. Like the penis, the clitoris contains erectile tissue so that when a woman gets sexually excited, the clitoris becomes engorged (filled) with blood and becomes twice the size as it is in its more relaxed state.

Most women need to have their clitoris stimulated in order to have an orgasm, but some can have orgasms through vaginal intercourse (the penis is almost always stimulated through vaginal intercourse, so orgasms are more common for men during this type of sex!). There is absolutely nothing wrong with a woman who can only have an orgasm through masturbation or stimulation of her clitoris by a partner—much like there is nothing wrong with a man who only has an orgasm through stimulation of his penis.

There is no one way for someone to have an orgasm, but there are some things that are common. First, people need to be comfortable with themselves and their partner (unless they are masturbating; then they are their own partner!). People also need to feel relaxed and comfortable with the surroundings. Genitals most likely need stimulation, and interruption of this stimulation can prevent a person from having an orgasm (but sometimes stopping and starting can feel good—it depends on the person). Finally, the most important thing is that all the people involved are enjoying themselves.

You might hear debates about clitoral and vaginal orgasms; some people try to say that one is better than the other, but the truth is an orgasm is an orgasm. The clitoris has more nerve endings than inside the vagina, so that's why some women have an easier time or can only have an orgasm if their clitoris is stimulated. But it's important to remember that so much of sexual attraction and responses comes from how a person feels. Therefore, whether a person orgasms or not has just as much to do with how that person is feeling emotionally as it does with what that person is experiencing physically. The more relaxed, happy, confident, and comfortable a person is, the more likely an orgasm will be a part of sexual activity.

But there are some differences between orgasms that are based in anatomy. Orgasms with penises are usually more obvious than clitoral ones because the ejaculation is more obvious. Also, after a penis ejaculates, it enters what is called a refractory period. This is a time of "recovery" where it becomes physically impossible for a penis to have an erection immediately after having an orgasm. Clitorises may want or need rest after an orgasm, but they don't experience this refractory period, which is why some clitorises are able to have multiple orgasms in a shorter period of time.

There is a lot of hype around orgasm, and it's hard to sort out the truth. Researchers try, but many things remain a mystery or a myth. For example, the jury is still out when it comes to female ejaculation—some people say it happens, while others do not. Same thing goes with the "G-spot." There are some people who swear by this special, extra sensitive area inside the vagina, and others who think it's a load of baloney.

Then there are others who wonder whether it's possible to have too much sexual pleasure. Here's one question and expert response on that topic:

Question:
Is it normal for your testicles to be sore after ejaculating a bunch of times in a short period of time, say three to five times in a day or two?
—Nineteen-year-old

Answer:
Yes, it's normal. After ejaculation, pelvic muscles and the muscles which move the testicles up and down have very strong contractions. These muscles may tend to ache if one ejaculates frequently. It's not dangerous, it just hurts.
Good Luck,
Dr. X, We Are Talking, teen health website

Going to the Doctor

Going to get your health checked—even if everything feels fine—is a normal part of life. Even though it is important for individuals to take care of their own sexual health, no one can do it alone. That's why it's recommended that young people between the ages of twelve and twenty-one get a well-visit checkup every year. Here are other reasons to go see a doctor about your reproductive and sexual health:

- You are sexually active and want to make sure everything is in working order.
- You are thinking of becoming sexually active and want to be safe and smart about it.
- You are concerned about a pregnancy.
- You want to see how things are doing "down there."
- You want birth control that requires a prescription.
- You want to talk about safer sex options with a professional.
- You experience pain in the pelvic region.
- You are experiencing an unusual discharge or bleeding in your genitals.

Getting these checkups can keep you healthy and possibly prevent any potential problems from getting worse (or developing in the first place).

Usually, people choose to go to a primary care or family doctor. There is also a type of doctor that specializes in the sexual health of uteruses, vaginas, and ovaries. This doctor is known as a gynecologist (or OBGYN, short for obstetrics and gynecology). Despite the stories you may hear, going to the doctor to get checked out is not that bad. And knowing what to expect before you go can make the experience that much easier. A routine exam consists of several parts. What parts you experience will depend on who you are, what you need, and the type of doctor you go to:

- *Getting the facts.* You will be asked to fill out a form or answer questions about your overall health, your sexual experiences, and any medications you take. Be honest. All the information you give is confidential, and telling the truth will give your doctor the right information to make decisions best for you.
- *A breast examination.* Although you are most likely a bit young to be concerned with breast cancer, a doctor will most likely massage your breasts to look for any unusual lumps. Hopefully, the doctor will also teach you how to do this yourself so that you can tell her if you feel anything out of the ordinary.
- *Pelvic examination.* Your doctor will check out the outside of your genitals. Then, for women, the doctor will use a speculum made of plastic or metal to open up your vagina and take a look inside. She will take a sample of your cervical mucus using a cotton swab (Q-Tip) or something that looks like a Popsicle stick. This may feel a little uncomfortable (the stretching and all), but it should not hurt. Ask your doctor for a mirror so that you can look inside your body and see what she sees. Then, your doctor will put some fingers into your vagina. She does this in order to see if your ovaries and uterus are doing okay.

The more you go to the doctor, the more it will feel like a normal part of life.

SEXUAL ORIENTATION AND GENDER IDENTITY

In a world where there are so many different people with different characteristics, it only makes sense that differences appear when it comes to gender and sexual attraction. While gender and sexual orientation are not choices people make, there are a lot of decisions to make when it comes to thinking about sexual and gender identities. People can make decisions about what to call themselves, how to express themselves, whether or not to come out, where to seek support, and how to advocate for the rights of people of all sexual orientations and gender identities. It's OK to feel whatever feelings you have about who you are attracted to and how you identify. There is no one right way to express your identity.

Definitions: Choosing Labels (or Not)

Sexual Orientation

Sexual orientation is the genders we are attracted to, both physically and romantically. You do not need to be in a relationship in order to identify with a sexual orientation. You can be in a situation where you have never been in a relationship before or have never been sexual with anyone. You can be in between relationships and still have a sexual orientation. There are many different sexual orientations. They include the following:

- Gay—men who are attracted to men
- Lesbian—women who are attracted to women
- Straight—women who are attracted to men, and men who are attracted to women
- Bisexual—people who are attracted to both men and women

- Pansexual—people who are attracted to people of all genders
- Asexual—people who don't feel attracted to any genders

There are many more sexual orientations than this, but this gives you a sense of the many ways people are attracted to others.

Sexual orientation is how a person feels inside. Sometimes a person may outwardly identify by a particular sexual orientation, while other times that person might decide to keep orientation quiet. When people publicly announce their own sexual orientations, those become their sexual identities. Sexual identity is how a person considers oneself to others when it comes to expressing sexual and/or romantic attractions to others. Culturally, "straight" people don't walk around announcing to the world whom they are attracted to, nor does anybody expect it of them. In the same way, people who do not identify as straight should not have to share that part of who they are. It's a personal choice as to whether to be public about your sexual orientation.

Similarly, some people may act on their sexual orientation—that is, have a relationship with or engage in sexual activities with another person in a way that matches their sexual orientation. However, there are many reasons why that may or may not happen. Some people may not find a suitable partner. Some may not feel safe to express their sexual identities in their communities or with their families. Others may find themselves attracted to someone who doesn't "match" their sexual orientation and decide to have a relationship with that person because it feels good. While for many people sexual orientation, sexual identity, and sexual behavior match each other, it's not the case for everyone.

Sexual orientation can stay the same throughout someone's life, or it can change over time. Some people like to think of sexual orientation as "fluid"; while no one can change your sexual orientation, your orientation may change over time as you grow and change. For example, one study found that over half of young adults aged eighteen to twenty-six years experienced changes in their sexual attractions.[1] The bottom line is this: your sexual orientation is yours and

More about Asexuality

- Not all people who identify as asexual have the same kinds of feelings. Some people who identify as asexual have romantic feelings toward other people, but not sexual feelings. Others will have sexual feelings toward another person, but only rarely or only when they are very much in love with someone. Some people who identify as asexual do not have any romantic or sexual feelings toward others.

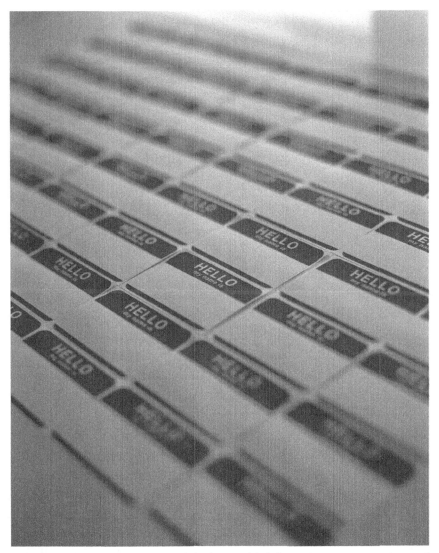

You get to choose whatever label you think best fits your gender and sexual preferences.

Movie Review (Cult Classic):
But I'm a Cheerleader
(1999, 1h 32m)

A popular cheerleader, Megan (Natasha Lyonne), is feared
to be lesbian by her parents, so she is shipped off to a camp designed to set her
"straight." There, she meets other gay and lesbian teens who struggle with accepting their sexual identity when everyone else wants them to just act "normal."

yours alone. No one should tell you what it is or should be. No one should tell you how you should label yourself, or if you should label yourself at all. These are your choices to make, and you can make them when you're ready to. And, as you learn more, you may decide you want to describe your sexual orientation in a different way; that's OK too. It's all part of the learning process.

In the same way, you should not define anyone else's sexual orientation. You should not label anyone by guessing based on their looks, behavior, or relationships status. You should respect a person's sexual orientation and identity, even if they do not make sense to you.

Gender Identity

Gender identity is how much you identify with being a man, woman, another gender, or no gender. The words *gender* and *sex* are sometimes used interchangeably, but they are different: *sex* is the word you use when you describe someone biologically—a person's hormones, anatomy, and chromosomes. *Gender* is different: gender is more about social roles and expectations.

When someone's biology "matches" the gender identity that was given at birth, we might say that person is cisgender. If someone's biology is different from the gender identity assigned at birth, that person might identify as transgender. When someone has a biological makeup that includes some characteristics of being male and some characteristics of being female, that person might identify as intersex. Within the identities of transgender and intersex, there are a spectrum of beliefs and feelings about how masculine and how feminine people feel, and how people may or may not wish to alter their bodies to align with their gender identities. But remember, just as it is with sexual orientation, a person can choose a gender identity that is comfortable and feels right, and whatever that choice is, others should respect it.

And just as people have a gender identity, they also have a gender expression. Gender expression is how people present themselves to the world through their appearance, behavior, dress, speech patterns, hobbies, and other things. A person's gender expression can be masculine, feminine, androgynous (having characteristics that are both masculine and feminine), or something else. Some people are gender nonconforming, which means they are perceived to have, or express, gender characteristics and/or behaviors that do not fit in the societal expectations of their biological sex.

While it's more common for a person to have a matching gender expression and gender identity, this is not always the case. People may not feel safe expressing themselves as the gender they are, or may not have the support they need to express themselves as the gender they wish to show the world. The bottom line is,

Pronouns

There are many different pronouns besides *he* and *she*. Some people use *ze, xe, per,* or *hu* to reflect that there are more than just two different genders. If you aren't sure what pronoun someone prefers, just ask (respectfully, of course!).

respect a person's gender identity by calling that person by the name that person chooses and using the pronoun (he, she, ze, etc.) that person chooses to go by.

Coming Out

For the most part, people go through life assuming that most people are heterosexual. This is because heterosexual (or straight) is the most common sexual orientation—but it's also because our society makes it easier for people who identify as heterosexual to exist in the world. People who wish to be more public about their sexual orientation may choose to come out to friends, family, and/or the community.

Deciding to reveal your sexual orientation or gender identity to others can be a pretty big deal. It can be an exciting time. It can possibly be a scary time. You might not be sure whether to tell others. You might feel like you are putting yourself on the line, making yourself vulnerable, and possibly opening yourself up to rejection from those who will not accept who you are. You might feel like you are being true to yourself and love the idea of being honest with yourself and those close to you. Here are some things to think about regarding whether to come out:

- Coming out means that you are no longer hiding a part of who you are. You might feel that you are a more authentic self.
- Make sure you have an ally. Even if that person is an online buddy, knowing you have someone you can talk to about the experience will help you feel strong.
- Ask yourself who you want to come out to. How accepting do you think this person will be? How much control does that person have over you? It's not a pleasant thought, but be honest with yourself. If you come out, do you think you will be kicked out of your home? Get a bad grade? Lose

Youth Speak Out: On Identity, by Kellyn, Age 16

Prior to entering high school, I never suspected that I could be anything other than a straight girl. A couple years later, neither of these labels apply to me anymore.

Realizing that I was bisexual was a shock to me as well as to a lot of people who knew me. It took me a long time to realize that I was crushing on another girl, but I eventually had to confront myself. "Well, you clearly like her. What does that mean for you?" I knew that I was still attracted to boys, and so I slipped fairly effortlessly into my new label. I am incredibly lucky to have a very inclusive and progressive high school and group of friends, so coming out at school was fairly easy. My family, however, is very religious, with values that are not accepting of many aspects of the LGBTQ community. Coming out to them was extremely hard for me because at the time I also had to tell them about struggles I was having with my mental health. We still disagree about most things surrounding sexuality and gender.

I started questioning my gender a while later, right before I began my junior year of high school. For a while I had no idea what was happening, and I didn't feel quite the same immediate support that I had when I had been questioning my sexuality. For a while I felt like I was drifting, researching gender identities and asking for help and opinions from my close friends. I went through a few different terms before I settled on agender, a non-binary gender identity.

I still struggle with deciding how and when to share this part of me with certain people. Even now I am still exploring my sexual and gender identity as well as how to express myself, but I believe that this is vital to my happiness and to being my best self.[a]

a friend? If so, don't blame yourself—it's not your fault at all. But it is important to think about your safety and security before coming out.

- Set aside a time to talk to the person. Being in a calm, quiet mood will help a lot when talking to someone about something as serious as this. Trying to rush this conversation will only make things tenser than they need to be. Coming out on social media may also not be the best idea because it's harder to control the conversation, and it makes it less personal.

- Be prepared for any reaction. The person you come out to might be happy, angry, proud, confused, excited, surprised, upset, or a combination of feelings. The person may act one way at first and another way later.
- Find a way to celebrate when you come out to someone! It takes a lot of courage to come out, and you should be proud of yourself for doing so.
- Remember that you are you. Let friends and family know that you are still the same person you have always been, with the same interests, feelings, and life—you are just letting them in on another part of the complex person you are.
- Don't feel pressured to come out. It's your choice and your choice alone. Come out only when you're ready and you want to.

Transitioning

Some trans people, in addition to coming out, may also want to begin transitioning to a different gender. Transitioning means changing one's gender expression so that it better matches gender identity. Transitioning can be done through clothing, voice tone, and makeup. It can also be done through altering one's body in medical and nonmedical ways. Depending on how old you are and what state you live in, you may be able to access certain medications that stop puberty so that your body does not develop sexual characteristics that do not match your gender identity. You may be able to take hormones to better align your body with your gender identity. Surgeries, however, are almost always only done on adults who have lived as the gender that matches their identity for at least a year.

Support

All people need support in their lives. When someone wishes to explore sexual orientation or gender identity, or wishes to come out to others, that person can't do it alone. The good news is that there are many places to go for support. In addition to talking to a friend, sibling, parent, or trusted adult, here are some other places to consider:

School/GSAs

About half of schools have a gay-straight alliance (GSA). GSAs are student-run organizations that bring together students of all sexual and gender orientations (even straight and cisgender students) in order to create a safe place in schools for young people to get together and work toward equality for everyone. Students in schools with GSAs are less likely to hear negative comments directed at LGBT (lesbian, gay, bisexual, trans) students, and are more likely to have teachers and staff intervene when they witness mistreatment of LGBT students.[2] If your school doesn't have a GSA but you would like to start one, visit the Gay Straight Alliance Network at gsanetwork.org to learn how!

Community Support

If you do not feel as though there is someone you know whom you can rely on, there may be a community group in your area that can help. There may be an LGBT community center near you, or some youth drop-in centers can be a good place to go. If you aren't sure where to start, try talking to someone at PFLAG. PFLAG is a national organization whose mission is to support LGBT youth, their families, and allies. Many chapters across the nation provide support groups, newsletters, and do advocacy work to achieve full equality for people who are LGBT. To find the location closest to you, or check out all their online resources, visit www.pflag.org.

Religious Institutions

Many assume that in order to be religious, you have to be straight and cisgender—that's not true. While some religious institutions are not as accepting of people of different sexual and gender orientations, there are some religions and places of worship that are more welcoming of all people. There are many LGBT-affirming religious leaders; they may be difficult to find at first, but being gay or trans does not mean that you cannot maintain your faith. The Religious Institute (religiousinstitute.org) is a multifaith organization that supports all people, no matter who they are, how they identify, or how they express themselves. Visiting the website may inform you as to how your religion understands different sexual and gender orientations. The truth is, many LBGT persons are able to continue practicing their faiths while remaining true to who they are.

Online Support

Although face-to-face contact with other young people of different sexual orientations and gender identities is important, sometimes that is not always possible. Smaller communities, and some areas of the United States in general, are less likely to have local resources for LGBT young people. In these cases, sometimes online technologies and mobile phones provide young people access to information and support that just don't exist elsewhere for them. Even if a young person has local support and resources, sometimes getting more information and support online is appealing because of the wealth of information available, and the relative anonymity one can have when online. This anonymity can give young people a chance to express themselves and explore. Young people find websites where they can feel accepted and find others like themselves to engage in discussion, read personal stories, and feel less isolated. Some online communities also offer more direct support and provide opportunities for advocacy. A great website to help you get started in finding information and support online is www.youth resource.com, a directory for all gay, lesbian, bisexual, transgender teens and their allies that's been created by young people for young people!

Advocacy

No matter your sexual orientation or gender identity, you can advocate for equal rights for all people. In our society, it's not as easy for those who aren't straight and cisgender to navigate through life. Biases and fears based on sexuality and gender are sometimes called homophobia (the fear of homosexuals) or transphobia (the fear of trans people). Homophobia and transphobia can be experienced in many ways:

- Name-calling or hearing derogatory words in random conversations
- Losing friends because of sexual orientation or gender identity
- Being considered different, wrong, sinful, strange, or mentally ill
- Violence
- Facing laws that discriminate based on sexual orientation and/or gender identity
- Bullying online and in person

Unfortunately, there are many examples of these types of mistreatment and discrimination. For example, as of 2015, over half of states didn't have any nondiscrimination policies in place to protect LGBT employees. One study found that most LGBT students were verbally harassed, and one in three were physically harassed. This discrimination and victimization experienced in school has serious consequences: lower grades, depression, and a smaller chance of going to college.[3]

There are many ways to advocate for sexual and gender equality, for example, simply being a friend who can be trusted, remembering that no matter which gender you fall in love with it can be just as exciting when it goes well and it can hurt just as much when things don't work out as expected, or offering true friendship and sharing your experiences are great ways to help anyone feel accepted. Seeing

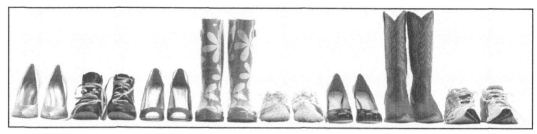

There is a lot of diversity within sexual orientation and gender identity.

In the News

In 2015, the Supreme Court ruled that the United States Constitution guarantees a right to same-sex marriage.

people as their whole selves, and not just their gender or sexual orientation, is also a way to show support because you are accepting people for who they are.

You can also advocate for someone by standing up for and with that person when you witness unfair treatment. First, don't engage in or tolerate name-calling. If you see a classmate being harassed or bullied because of sexual orientation or gender identity—whether it's known or just assumed—there are many things you can do. You can intervene directly when it's safe: stand up for the person being harassed, or challenge people who use derogatory words ("fag" or "that's so gay"). You can talk to a trusted adult or friend about what you witnessed and together find resources to support the person being bullied.

When the bullying happens at school, check to see what antibullying policies your school has in place (if your school doesn't have any, maybe it's time to work toward some!). If you see a teacher ignoring (or even encouraging) any form of homophobic or transphobic behavior, let the principal know. If you are still being ignored, put your complaint in writing and send the letter to both the principal and the school board. The American Civil Liberties Union has resources about how to fight discrimination if things get serious. Bullying and harassment should not happen to anyone, and you can almost always do something to help stop it.

Finally, there are sometimes opportunities to become more politically involved in fighting for LGBT rights. Advocates for Youth and Lamba Legal are two places to start to get involved on a national level.

CHOOSING NOT TO HAVE SEX

Choosing not to have sex (many call it practicing abstinence) is a great choice for many young people. It's the most effective way of protecting yourself from an STD (sexually transmitted disease) or unexpected pregnancy. It's a wonderful way to focus on other priorities in your life. Sometimes people choose not to have sex until they have a better understanding of what they want out of sex and/or a relationship. When you choose not to have sex, you need to consider two things:

1. What activities you consider sex, and therefore will refrain from
2. How long you will not do those activities

We are going to talk about these two parts of your decision to abstain from sex so that it's easier to understand both why this choice is right for you (or not right for you) and why some people may choose it but not others. This chapter may also help those who choose not to have sex stick to their decision despite all the pressures out there for people to have sex.

What Is Sex?

In order to decide if you are ready to, or want to, have sex, it's a good idea to know what sex is. Don't laugh. There are a lot of people in this world, and almost all of them have a different idea of what it means to have sex. Sometimes, these different ideas as to what sex is and isn't come up in considering whether one is a virgin or not. Basically, a virgin is someone who has not had sex before. But what does that mean, really? Is a person who has never had vaginal intercourse but has had oral sex a virgin? Is a person who has experimented with cybersex still a virgin? Is a person who started to have sex, but lost the erection before ejaculation still a virgin? Different people may have different answers to these scenarios. The concept of virginity is not as clear as you might think.

Along the same line of thinking, people who choose not to have sex sometimes say that they are practicing abstinence. Again, this seems like a clear enough decision. If someone wants to be abstinent, then all the person has to do is choose not to have sex. But how clear-cut is this decision? According to the dictionary, to "abstain" from something means "to refrain deliberately and often with an effort of self-denial from an action or practice."[1] So does that mean if someone decides to not have sex, that individual needs a lot of "effort" and is engaging in "self-denial"? That sort of talk makes abstinence sound hard or even impossible! And we know that is not true. Many people do not have sex and feel completely fine and comfortable with their decision. Indeed, they feel deep down that it's the right thing for them to do. Other people choose not to have sex, and it is a difficult decision and they have to work harder to stay true to their decision. Either way, it's a decision made for reasons that are different for each person. I don't like to think of the term *abstinence* as a bad thing, and I certainly don't like that dictionary definition! Instead, I like to think of people who abstain from sex as people who are choosing not to have sex. They are making a personal decision. They are proud of their behavior and satisfied with their decision.

So, if a person decides to be abstinent, which sexual behaviors are "allowed" or "not allowed"? Can a person receive oral sex from someone else and be abstinent? Have anal sex? Give someone a hand job? Once again, a concept that seems so clear becomes a bit fuzzy when you think about it. Again, there are different possible answers to these questions, and no answer is more right than another. It's up to an individual to make a personal decision first, and then discuss that choice with a partner, if relevant.

First, it's important to define virginity and abstinence for yourself, and then stick to your definition and stay true to your choices and boundaries. Only you can decide what is right for you, comfortable for you, and best for you. These are the definitions of sex, abstinence, and virginity that matter the most—the ones that are thought out carefully by you.

Remember, no matter what your definitions of virginity and abstinence are, defining these words is helpful not only for you, but also to anyone you have sex with. Why, you may ask, should you share your ideas of virginity and abstinence with a sexual partner? There are many reasons: so that you and your partner can protect and honor both of your sexual beliefs; so you two can be sexually healthy; so you can make sure the two of you are consenting to anything that may happen. For example, say that you believe that someone who has had oral sex is no longer a virgin, but your partner believes that someone who has had oral sex and not vaginal sex is still a virgin. Not a big deal, you say—just a difference of opinion. Think again. A person who has had oral sex is at risk for having an STD; translation, your partner, who believes he or she is a virgin, potentially has an STD. The proper STD prevention may not take place between the two of you, and the disease could be spread. A little communication about beliefs and practices can go a long way in taking care of each other, your health, and the relationship.

Think about it: What do you think sex is? What does it mean to be abstinent? What does it mean if you choose not to have sex? Really take the time these questions deserve. It might even help to write them down somewhere private. Revisit your ideas every so often to see if your beliefs change over time as you learn more about your sexuality.

Defining Abstinence

A group of young people were asked which sexual activities were a part of being abstinent. Table 3.1 shows what some of them said.

Table 3.1. Sexual Activities and Perceptions of Abstinence

Activity	Percent Who Said It Was a Part of Abstinence
Deep kissing	92%
Touching their own genitals to orgasm	49%
Touching their own genitals without orgasm	60%
Performing oral sex to orgasm	41%
Receiving oral sex with no orgasm	44%

Source: E. Sandra Byers, Joel Henderson, and Kristina M. Hobson, "University Students' Definitions of Sexual Abstinence and Having Sex," *Archives of Sexual Behavior* 38 (2009): 665–674.

See why you can't assume someone's definition of abstinence is the same as yours? Talk to your partner!

The History of Abstinence

Some cultures past and present believe that young people should lose their virginity as part of a coming-of-age ceremony. The ancient Greeks didn't think it was such a good idea to marry a virgin; the men wanted to know if a woman was capable of having sex before they married her. It wasn't until the rise of Christianity that virginity was considered more important. Today, there are mixed opinions as to whether someone should remain a virgin until marriage.[a]

How Long Will You Wait?

Now that you have thought about how you wish to define sex and, therefore, abstinence—you have personally decided what you will and will not do when choosing not to have sex—we need to tackle the second part: how long you will be abstinent; how long you will choose not to have sex. If you choose not to have sex, you have to ask yourself, "For how long am I choosing not to have sex?"

There are many time frames in which people will choose not to have sex. Some people will choose not to have sex for their entire lives; people such as priests and nuns make this sort of decision. So do people who identify as asexual. Other people choose not to have sex until they reach a certain time in their life—marriage, graduation from high school, or until they are a certain age. Others wait until a certain situation comes along—they fall in love, they truly trust a person, they feel mature enough to handle being sexual with another person. Finally, there are those who simply choose not to have sex because of logistics—there is no condom at this time, they are drunk and want to make a decision to have sex when their head is clearer, they are in a public place. As you can see from these examples, some people are choosing not to have sex for a short amount of time, while others are waiting a little bit longer. The point is that it's important to wait to have sex until you are in a safe and comfortable situation—and your partner feels the same way. Everyone has a different length of time that they will choose to be abstinent. It's important to decide what length of time is right for you and your partner. No sex should happen without consent from everyone involved (see chapter 8 for more about this important topic).

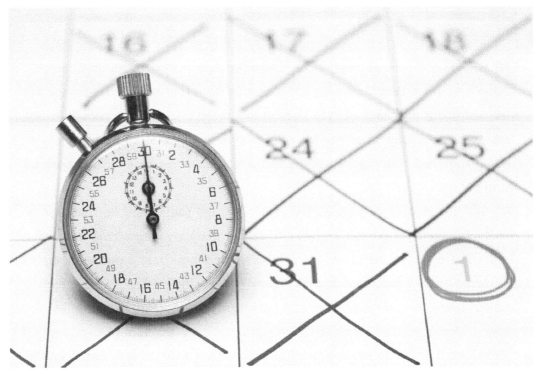

Everyone has a different timetable for being abstinent.

Just as there are many different lengths of time to wait, there are also many different reasons to wait. Here are just a few:

- You want to get to know your partner better.
- You want to concentrate on school.
- You want to follow your religious beliefs.
- You want to learn more about safer sex.
- You're not in a private location.
- You don't feel ready.
- Your gut tells you to wait.

What reasons do you have for waiting?

Practicing Abstinence

Choosing not to have sex does not mean that you cannot be sexual. There is a big difference between having sex and engaging in sexual behaviors. What I mean is *abstinence is not anti-sex!* This may surprise you at first. But, if you think about it, most people have sexual feelings, and there are so many ways to express one's

Youth Speak Out: Why I'm Waiting, by Brad

My whole life I've never really been interested in a sex life or putting time into actually knowing what love means. My parents have told me the basics, and I've learned things in school, but I'm just not interested or don't care enough to ask more. I don't usually have time for girlfriends or any of that because usually I'm doing a sport or training for a sport and when I have free time I like to spend it with my best friends.

Sex and love are a huge part in people's lives. You should do that type of stuff with the right person. I'm already seeing people younger than me having sex with a bunch of people and even getting pregnant. They even have a reality TV show *16 and Pregnant* on MTV. That's just a huge part of being a teen in school taken away because now you have to focus on being a parent. I'm not saying I won't have sex later, but for now I could care less about sex and love. I am gonna start taking advantage of being a kid because I'm only gonna be this age once and I wanna make it count. In my opinion I think I'm still too young to have sex or even think about it. It may not be too young for other people; if they think they are ready, then cool, but I'm not ready for that experience yet and I want to save something that important for the right person that I think I'm gonna be with for a really long time.[b]

sexuality that it is possible to not do some sexual activities, but still have plenty to choose from if you want. Let's think about some things that people might do with another person (with full consent of course) and still remain abstinent.

There are many things you can do that can be very sexual and intimate, without having sex. Generally, there are two kinds of sexual behaviors—those that involve touching and those that do not. Here are some examples of things that involve touch:

- Kissing someone on the lips, neck, or back
- Being kissed on the hand or ear
- Touching someone so lightly that they can barely feel it
- Exchanging massages
- Holding someone close

And here are some examples of things that do not involve touch:

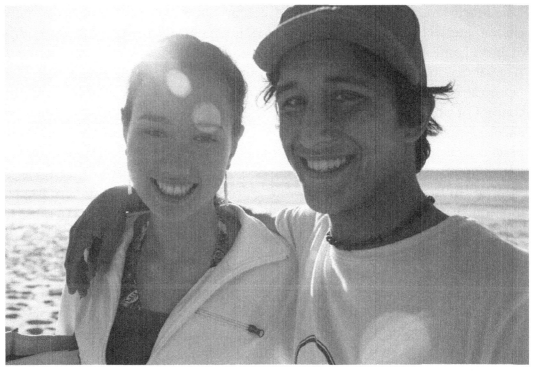

There are many great ways to show someone how much you like them without having sex.

- Exchanging flirty, sexy, mushy, loving texts
- Blowing in someone's ear
- Sending a surprise gift
- Making slow, caring eye contact

Pretty cool list, huh? Feel free to add to it or take away from it, depending on your definition of abstinence and what your partner does and does not like. The point is, you can express your feelings for someone and still be abstinent. And that person can express feelings for you and respect your boundaries. Just remember, different people have different definitions of abstinence and all should be respected. But in the end, people who say that abstinence is "no fun" just might be lacking understanding or imagination.

Abstinence as Safer Sex

As we've already discussed, there are many different types of sexual activities that people may or may not consider to be sex. However, in this section we are going to be focusing on abstinence as a way to avoid unplanned pregnancy, so the type of sex I am focusing on here is vaginal intercourse. As many of you have heard several times from many different places (school, the news, parents, church, etc.), choosing not to have vaginal intercourse is the most effective form of birth control. We hear this over and over again because it's a true statement. If a person does not have vaginal intercourse, there will be no pregnancy. That person also will have a lower chance of getting an STD. But as all things are, this concept of abstinence as safer sex is not as simple as you may think. In order for choosing not to have vaginal intercourse to be 100 percent effective, it has to be practiced correctly—that means it has to be done each and every time you are in a sexual situation. It's easy to see that the best of intentions sometimes do not go as planned. In fact, studies show that young people who choose not to have vaginal intercourse do not always follow through on their plans. Up to 25 percent of teens who say they are not having vaginal intercourse actually change their minds (or at least their behaviors) and do have it after all.[2] So what does this mean? It means that choosing not to have vaginal intercourse can fail as a method of contraception, just like all the other contraceptive methods reviewed in chapter 6. Used "correctly"—that is, if the person truly does not have vaginal intercourse—no pregnancy will occur. But used "incorrectly"—in other words, if a person has vaginal intercourse even if it wasn't planned—then a pregnancy can happen if a backup method is not used.

Here's summary of the abstinence method:

How it works: A person chooses not to engage in vaginal intercourse—the one behavior that will cause pregnancy.

What makes it a good choice: If done properly, it's 100 percent effective against pregnancy and helps lower the risk of STDs.

Why it might not be right for you: You may want to have vaginal intercourse.

How to get it: You make the decision and do your best to keep it.

Cost: Free!

Wait time until it works: There's no wait; it works right away.

How well does it work: It works as well as the people involved with each other follow through with the decision.

What can go wrong: Something happens that makes a person have vaginal intercourse even when he or she chose not to.

SEX AND SAFER SEX: WHAT IS IT? WHO'S DOING IT? AND OTHER IMPORTANT QUESTIONS

••

Y ou feel that everyone is having sex; you feel like you are the only one not having sex; you feel as though you should be having sex. There is all this talk in
the news, on TV, in schools about how young people are having sex. The cover-
age on the issue is to the point where it can feel as though all teens are having sex
all the time. This is far from the truth. Fact is, by eleventh grade, about half of
young people report having sex.[1] The level of sexual experience of young people
has stayed pretty consistent over the past ten years (and is lower than it was in the
1990s), even though the media (and many adults) make it sound like young people
are having more sex than ever before. In addition, young people who are having
sex are using contraception more often than they were in the 1990s, meaning that
they are acting more responsibly than their parents when they are choosing to
have sex. Not surprisingly, because young people are having more responsible sex,
their pregnancy rate is lower, too.

No matter what others think, whether you are or are not having sex, you are
not alone. No matter what you are doing, choosing to have or not to have sex,
there are others making the same decisions as you are. Even when it comes to
kissing, experiences differ. While it's true that most teens have kissed someone
before (nine out of ten say they have), when it comes to deep kissing, 80 percent
say they have done it.[2] That may sound like a lot, but if you flip the percentage
around that means one in five teens has not French kissed. That's a lot of people
who have never done it.

Also, different people tend to do different things when it comes to sex. For example, white teens tend to have more oral sex than African American and Hispanic youth. African American youth, on average, have sex earlier than other races and ethnicities, while Asian teens tend to have sex later on in life.[3] These are generalizations to be sure—different individuals in these racial groups will have different experiences—but there are trends such as these that researchers look at.

What Is Sex? The Health Perspective

Even though you already thought about a personal definition of sex after reading the previous chapter, I am going to bring in a specific definition of sex now. Since this chapter focuses on safer sex, I will define what sex is by one of the reasons people choose not to have sex—for health reasons. For this case, I use the definition of sex that the Centers for Disease Control and Prevention (CDC) uses when it talks about how to best prevent sexually transmitted diseases (STDs).[4] In a nutshell, sex is connecting any two of the following body parts:

- Penis
- Vagina
- Vulva
- Clitoris
- Anus
- Mouth

As you can see, there are many possible body part combinations; therefore, there are many ways that STDs can be transmitted—via the mouth, genitals, or anus. According to the CDC, these types of sexual contact all "count" as sex because they can spread sexually transmitted diseases.

What Is Safer Sex?

If you want to do everything you possibly can to not face an unexpected pregnancy or STD, there are three choices you can make:

1. Choose not to have sex.
2. Use a condom.
3. Along with your partner, get tested for STDs and then both of you remain monogamous—that means, stay with each other and only each other.

> ### Defining Abstinence
> • If you are choosing to be abstinent—that is, if you are choosing not to have sex—I strongly suggest that you use the CDC definition of sex, too. That way, you and anyone you are with have a better chance of staying healthy.

In this chapter, we will spend some time looking at the third option. Condoms are discussed in chapter 6, and choosing not to have sex was covered in the previous chapter.

Being Safe through Testing and Monogamy

There are two parts to this safer sex strategy. The first part is to make sure you and your partner do not have any STDs in the first place, and then once the coast is clear, the two of you need to be monogamous and stay monogamous so that you do not put yourself at risk for getting an STD from someone else.

Part One: Getting Tested for STDs

The *only way* to know if you have an STD is to get tested for STDs. The only way you are going to know if your partner has an STD is for your partner to get tested. After that, both of you need to trust each other to tell the truth about the results. No matter the outcome, it's important to be honest.

Where to Go?

There are a few different places where you can go to get tested for STDs: a doctor's or nurse's office, a mobile van, a school-based health center, and a clinic. There are differences among all of these choices, and not all the choices are available close to everyone. One important thing to consider when getting tested for STDs is whether the place you go has confidential or anonymous testing. What is the difference between an anonymous and a confidential test? A confidential test is like a secret—someone promises to keep something secret, but there is a way to find out the facts. A confidential test means that although no one is supposed to tell the results of your test, your name is attached to test results and it goes on a record. On the other hand, an anonymous test means you can use a fake name or number to identify yourself so that no one but you can link you to the test results. So, if it's important for you to have your test results be anonymous, and not just confidential, look for a place that offers anonymous testing. Clinics can often provide such services, but not all clinics give anonymous tests, so ask before you assume anything.

Here are some other possible differences and considerations when it comes to STD testing sites. Think about which are important to you and ask before you make an appointment.

- *Insurance possibilities and problems:* You may be covered under your insurance, but parents may see a bill.
- *Cost:* Sometimes clinics can be the cheapest option, especially if you don't have health insurance.
- *Trust:* Who do you trust more? A doctor? Nurse? Testing done at a clinic? Only you can decide.
- Scheduling: Some places are easier to get an appointment than others.
- *Counseling:* Find out if the place you get tested has counseling services too—an extra bonus!
- *Contraceptives:* Some places have free condoms or are able to prescribe birth control while some places cannot.

What Will Happen When I Get There?

There are a few different ways to get tested for STDs—it depends on what STD you want to be tested for. Sometimes all a health-care provider needs to do is take a swab of the infected area (genitals, anus, or mouth) in order to get a cell sample. Sometimes you just have to pee in a cup. There are a few cases (some HIV and herpes tests) require a blood sample. Talk to your health-care provider about what sexual activities you have engaged in, and the two of you can have a conversation about which STD tests make the most sense to do.

When you go to a clinic to get an HIV test or other STD blood test, a trained medical professional will take a sample of blood from your arm, tell you when the results of your test will be ready (usually a week or two), and then let you go home. Be sure to ask if you need to come back to the clinic to get your test results or if you are able to get them by calling. If you can, it's always a good idea to get your test results in person, because that way you can ask questions and get help right away if you need to. If the test is anonymous (remember, that means no one knows who you really are), you will either give a fake name or get an ID code when you call to make an appointment. This name or code will be the only name by which people know you. You may be asked to fill out some forms or surveys, but at no point should anyone ask you to put your actual name on them. Then,

SEX AND SAFER SEX **49**

after the test is done, you may get a slightly different ID code in order to get the results, or you will use the same code or name as the first time. The people at the clinic will let you know.

When you have a sample taken, the cells are put on a slide or in a tube and analyzed in a laboratory. If you gave a urine sample, that is also analyzed in a lab. As with blood tests, it takes a while to get the results, so be sure to ask when the results will be available.

Part Two: Staying Monogamous and Trusting Your Partner Will Do the Same

You got the first done—you and your partner were tested for STDs and, after any necessary treatments, you now know with confidence that you are both STD free! Excellent work. So, now you two can have sex forever and ever with each other and not worry about catching anything— right? Not quite. The two of you now have to trust each other and yourselves enough to know that you will not be sexual with anyone else except each other. Remember—you do not necessarily have to have sex to get an STD (herpes, for example, can be passed mouth to mouth)—so being with only one partner for any sort of sexual contact is a must for this to work. Talk to your partner. Know your partner. Listen to yourself and trust your instincts. If your partner is not even willing to get tested for STDs in the first place, that is a good sign that this is not a good safer sex method for the

Love and Trust

Love and trust may often go hand in hand, but they are *not* the same thing. You can love someone you do not trust (like when your baby brother plays with your cell phone), and you can trust someone you do not love (like a doctor or a teacher). So, just because you love someone, or are in love with someone, does not mean that you necessarily trust that someone to stay monogamous or to be STD-free if that person has not been tested. Don't let someone manipulate you by saying, "Why do we need to use a condom? Don't you love me?" If it's true, you can smile back and say that indeed you love that person, but you love you and your life as well and want to play it safe for now.

> **Don't Forget the Contraception!**
>
> Remember, you still have to use contraception when you have vaginal intercourse if you do not want a pregnancy to happen! That's what birth control pills, cervical caps, and all those other methods discussed in chapter 6 are for!

two of you. If you know your partner has cheated in the past (maybe that is even how the two of you started going out in the first place), then maybe this method is not the right one for you—at least not for a very long time. Remember, you could literally be putting your life into someone's hands by having unprotected sex. Be choosy about who that person is.

What Choice Are You Going to Make?

You are now aware of the three healthy and safer sex choices that are available to you. To recap, they are:

1. Choosing not to have sex
2. Using a condom (if you want to know more about using condoms, skip ahead to chapter 6 before reading the rest of this section)
3. Getting tested (both you and your partner) and staying monogamous

Which choice is best for you? Close your eyes, think about it, and decide. Then, say it out loud. And write it down. The more actively involved you are in making this decision, the more likely you are to stick with it. Next, choose a backup. What is your second choice on the list? If you opted for choice 2 for your first strategy, but no condoms are available, then what are you going to do? Having both a plan A and a plan B helps ensure that you will have a happier, healthier life. By choosing a plan and a backup plan, you are miles ahead of not only most people your age, but most older adults, too.

How Do You Feel about Sex?

You have the facts about safer sex. That's one part of the equation when it comes to deciding to have sex, but it's certainly not the only part. It's also important to consider your feelings about sex. Deciding whether to have sex is not a group decision; your parents, friends, favorite television show, or celebrity crush might influence your sexual decisions, but none of these should have the final say in your decision. The decision to have sex is a decision two people—and only two—make together. What you should figure out before you have sex—whether it be the first time or the next time—is whether you and your partner want to have sex. The way to know if your partner wants to have sex is to ask that person (see chapter 8 for information about consent). And although it may sound a bit weird, the way to find out if you want to have sex is to ask yourself. Really. On a day or night when you are by yourself, take some quality time to think about how you feel about sex and other sexual behaviors. It will probably take more time than just this one session to really understand how you feel about sex, and to figure out when and under what circumstances you would and would not want to have sex with someone, but starting with just this one time is a great start. The more you think about it, the more you will know who you are as a sexual being, and what your values are when it comes to engaging in different sexual activities. Not sure where to start? Here are some questions you can ask yourself to get started:

- Is it OK to kiss someone I just met that day?
- What sexual activities do I want to do the first time I hook up with someone?
- What do I think is the best age for me to start having sex?
- What sexual activities do I enjoy?
- What sexual activities do I find unappealing?
- Do I consider having oral sex as having sex?
- Under what circumstances would I send a sext to someone?

You can answer these questions in your head, or you can write out your answers in a journal or secret blog. Sometimes putting something in writing makes it more real, so you might want to try it. Also, these questions are not meant to be the only questions you should ask yourself. It's a good idea to think about other questions you have for yourself, write them down, and take the time to answer them. Then, go back to your questions and answers every so often to see if you feel the same way. You can also add questions and answers as they come up in your life. Questions that you come up with on your own are often a lot more meaningful than any questions you are going to find in a book.

Don't be worried if you do not know the answers to some questions right away. But if you are struggling to come up with answers, here's a suggestion: try to avoid answering the question in the moment. What that means is, if you are not sure what sexual activities you want to do the first time you hook up with

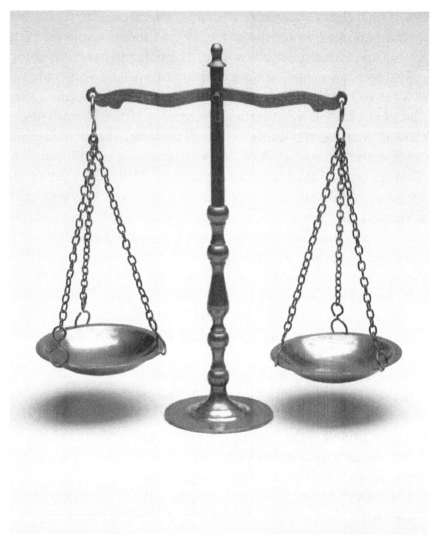

It's important to take the time to think about your sexual values.

someone, it's a good idea to not hook up with someone until you have an answer. Finding out by doing can lead to regretting things you have done because you didn't think about them carefully first. Take time to think about who you are as a sexual being and what you think you may or may not like—you're worth it. It's OK to wait to have sex, if that is what you want to do or if you're simply not sure what you want.

Are You Ready?

Many of you want to know an answer to a very difficult question: How do I know when I am ready to have sex? Well, that question, like all difficult questions, has no one answer. Everyone is different, and each time you consider having sex is a different situation that requires reflection. However, here is a list of things that I think you should be able to do before you have sex with someone:

- You know for sure that both you and the person you are with want to have sex.
- You and your partner feel no doubt about what you are doing.
- You and your partner do not feel ashamed about what you are doing.
- You and your partner feel comfortable talking about sexuality with each other.
- You and your partner have taken care of pregnancy and STD prevention, including knowing the STD status of you and your partner.
- You and your partner are ready and willing to have sex without having drugs or alcohol.
- You are being totally honest with your partner about your feelings, and you believe that your partner is being totally honest with you.
- You like your partner's friends and like the way your partner is around them.
- You are able to be yourself around your partner's friends.
- After you have sex, you will not feel the need to either hide the fact of what you did, nor feel the need to tell everyone what you did. Having sex is a private matter between you and your partner.
- You and your partner have discussed what you would do if there is a pregnancy (if there is a chance for pregnancy).
- You really want to have sex, because you want to, not just because your partner wants to.
- Your partner really wants to have sex, not just because you want to.

Long list, huh? You bet it is. Deciding to have sex is a very big deal and deserves to have a long checklist associated with it.

The Naked Dance

Another way to decide whether you are ready to have sex is to take yourself through the following mind exercise I like to call the Naked Dance: Could you do the Hokey-Pokey, Macarena, or some other silly dance, naked, in front of your partner (not while high or drunk)? If you can do this and have a good time doing it, you may be ready to have sex. Why? Well, doing a silly dance naked in front of your partner means a lot of things. It means:

- You are willing to be vulnerable in front of your partner.
- Your partner is willing to have fun with you during a vulnerable time.

- You are able to laugh at yourself, and you and your partner are able to laugh together while sharing an intimate moment.
- You are comfortable with your body.
- You trust that your partner will not tell the whole school about what you did.

All those things count for a lot! They show comfort and trust within yourself and between you and your partner. Those are good qualities to have when thinking about being sexual.

The First Time

You have thought about it on your own. You have talked about it with your partner. The two of you, both together and individually, are ready. You want to have sex together. Having sex for the first time comes with a very strange contradiction. Although very few people find it as special or loving or dramatic as they imagine it will be, having sex for the first time is an event you will remember. You will remember where you were, how it felt, when it happened, and of course who it was with. So take your first time seriously.

You have heard many things about "the first time," and most likely all of them are true—for those cases. This is because different people have different experiences when it comes to first times. One study asking young people about their first times found that the most common feelings were happiness, excitement, it was fun, nervousness, fear, and indifference (feeling "OK"). Many people had more than one of these feelings at the same time.[5] A first sexual experience is a mix of feelings, some more positive than others. That's normal. Sex can be an intense experience for many people. Sex also has a lot of baggage that comes along with it, thanks to the many different ways it is perceived in society—as a treasure, a gift to give to another, a "must-do," a "must get," the best thing ever, the thing that drives life purpose. Heavy stuff.

Despite all these different feelings and perceptions about having sex for the first time, there are some things that are true for everyone:

- A pregnancy can happen the first time someone has vaginal sex. It doesn't matter whether the sex lasts three seconds or a whole hour. If there is penetration, there is a chance of pregnancy, even if neither person orgasms (of course, ejaculation increases the chances substantially).
- It is possible to get an STD the first time a person has sex. Once again, the length of time or whether there are orgasms does not matter. If one person in the couple is infected, there is a chance the other person can become infected.

Youth Speak Out: Listing the Pros and Cons of Having Sex, by Sofie, Age 15

When deciding whether or not to have sex with someone, sometimes writing a list of pros and cons can be useful. The pros and cons should be considered for both people in the relationship.

First, you should ask yourself these questions: Will having sex benefit both of us? Is this just for sex or for love? If we are having sex and using a condom, what if it broke? Would my partner leave? When we have sex, will my partner spread rumors about me or what we did? Do I really want to go through with this? Do they?

Even writing out a table on a piece of paper can be helpful. Really think about the decision because it's important. Here's an example I made. This table can vary depending on the person who is writing it and what they do and do not like.

Pros	Cons
Could be a learning and fun experience	Could be a dull or bad experience
Could make the relationship better	The partner could break up with you, or you with them
Reliable and trustworthy person	Rumors might be spread
Could feel happy afterwards	Could feel guilty afterwards[a]

- The first time you have sex will shape your views about sex. Choose a good partner to share it with. Sure, there may be some mistakes and awkward moments, but with an understanding partner, those "imperfections" will make your experience unique. Some of you may not have chosen your first "sexual" experience due to abuse. While this experience will most likely shape your views about sex and sexuality, with support you can create more positive views of intimacy. See chapter 9 for more on sexual violence and recovery.
- The first time will not be as you expected it to be. This is because sex is unpredictable. Feelings are hard to figure out, messes happen, lots can go right and wrong. Keep talking to your partner, check in with yourself and each other, and have fun.

Here are some things that differ from couple to couple regarding having sex for the first time:

- *How long it lasts:* Many first times last only a few seconds. Others last longer because it may take a while for a body to be ready for sex. A penis needs to be hard enough for a condom to fit properly; a vagina needs to be wet enough for penetration to feel good. Mutual masturbation with lubricant can help or be a satisfying experience in itself.
- *How it feels:* Some barely feel a thing—rarely does a woman have an orgasm the first time she has sex with a man. Others feel great pleasure; still others, intense pain. The basic rule of thumb is, if it hurts a lot, try again later. Later can either mean in a couple of minutes after more kissing and other fun takes place, or another day, or another year. Some females' first times having vaginal intercourse are painful, either because the vagina is not wet enough for penetration, her muscles are too tense, or her hymen is stretching. Any of these sources of pain and discomfort can be solved by making sure she feels relaxed, is aroused enough, and feels comfortable with what she is doing. Nervousness is a very normal part of having sex, but feeling unsafe or uncomfortable is not. If it feels wrong, it is wrong. Make sure to check in with your partner to make sure things are still OK.
- *How the person feels afterward:* Some people feel great, others feel dreamy, and unfortunately, some don't feel so good after sex. Many have mixed feelings. Check in with yourself to see how you are feeling. Ask your partner, too. Talk about all the feelings you are both having. Once the sex is done, there is still plenty of sharing to do to bring you closer together.
- *Whether one or both of you orgasm:* Depending on the sexual activity, it's very possible that only one person will orgasm during the experience. In many sex activities, the focus is on one person's pleasure so it makes sense that this is the case. Don't worry about having orgasms at the same time, or at all. Orgasm may or may not be important to your partner. Check in with each other to see what's important, and how each person's desires can be respected.
- *Whether it will help or hurt the relationship:* Sex is a funny thing. No matter what, sex will change a relationship. For better or for worse depends on the couple and the individuals within the couple. If the sex is planned and discussed, and honest feelings are shared before and after the experience, chances are the relationship will grow closer. But if things are left unsaid and not everyone's feelings are acknowledged, the relationship could take a turn for the worse.

Question:

I had sex for the first time a couple of days ago. I bled fairly badly, and it continued to bleed, off and on for a day or two more. Is this normal?

—Seventeen-year-old in Massachusetts

Answer:

Light bleeding for a couple of days after first sex can be because the hymen, a piece of tissue in the vagina, has been ruptured, or there was some minor tearing. This is normal and should not be worried about. It can also be that there is not enough lubrication, causing small tears in the vaginal area. You can use a little water-based lubricant for extra lubrication, or use

Concerns about the "First Time"

Having sex for the first time can be a big deal, and many young people have a lot of questions about it. Here are some questions that were asked on my advice board:

- Can my doctor tell if I have had sex? Will he tell my parents?
- I had sex for the first time and did not orgasm; is there something wrong with me?
- My boyfriend and I had sex for the first time, and when I woke up the next day there was blood on my underwear! Should I worry about this or get it checked?
- During sex, do you also kiss the person you are with?
- How will I feel before and after sex?
- How bad will it hurt the first time I have sex? Will we have to stop because of the pain?

Oftentimes, there is no one answer to questions like this. But asking questions is a great way to start finding answers so that you are comfortable about having sex.

prelubricated condoms. As always, if you are concerned, or if it happens again, see your doctor.

I know you did not ask, but if you haven't already, please see a doctor (or clinic) to get a reliable method of birth control and use a condom every time you have vaginal or oral intercourse to protect against sexually transmitted infections. Good Luck!

Dr. X, We Are Talking, teen health website[6]

Casual Sex

Hookups, friends with benefits, flings—being sexual outside of a relationship happens for sure, but there isn't that much information about casual sex and young people. However, it's worth mentioning. Either through personal experiences or the rumor mill, you hear of people randomly hooking up at a party and going "all the way." Well, what are those experiences like? Are they fun? Safe? A good idea? What makes the casual hookup so seemingly popular? Some numbers may help us paint a picture of casual sex among young people. In one college, about half of the sexual experiences reported were not with a romantic partner. However, among those who had sex with a more casual partner, those experiences were with friends, not strangers. Also, 65 percent said that either drugs or alcohol were involved.[7] In another study with college students, of those who did have casual sex, less than half said they would do it again if they had the chance. However, more than half said they did not regret the experience.[8]

So what does this all mean? It looks like casual sex isn't uncommon, but it's certainly not universal. It also seems to leave people with mixed feelings, since less than half would repeat the experience if given the chance, but more than half have no regrets. The high rates of drugs and alcohol use mean that consent may

Movie Review: Friends with Benefits (2011; 1h 49m)

Jamie (Mila Kunis) and Dylan (Justin Timberlake) are friends, who then start hooking up and agree not to get emotionally involved with each other. But after dates with other people while trying to remain "just friends," the two realize that they do love each other.

not have been obtained properly (see chapter 8). So, is casual sex a good idea? Only you and the other person you are with can decide.

The Intimacy Approach to Sex

You've heard it before, but I will say it again—young people are given mixed messages about sex. On the one hand, they are told to "just say no" to sex, while on the other hand, they are bombarded with glorifying sexual images from the media and are often given the message that sex makes them more mature. Sex, in many ways, is considered the "be all end all" in relationships, and may even be considered the reason to be in a relationship in the first place—at least that is what so many of those beer commercials would have you believe.

But guess what? There is a lot more to a relationship than just having sex. In fact, it's more than possible to have a great relationship with someone, and not even have sex with that person. It's also possible to have a pretty crummy relationship with someone, even if you are having sex. In this section, we are going to look at the differences between sex and intimacy. In fact, I am going to make the point that if the goal of a relationship is to be intimate with another person, then that relationship will be a lot healthier for everyone involved.

Intimacy is a feeling of warmth and togetherness. An intimate relationship is a close, mature relationship that may or may not include sex. Most people do not see intimacy as the goal of a relationship or even a fun evening—they think sex should be the end result. When people come up to you after a party and ask, "So, did you get any last night?" they are not talking about cuddling, kissing, and "quality time." They are talking about sex. So if you answer, "Yeah, I really got to know this person really well and I think I actually like her! We talked about our families and then spent about half an hour tracing messages on each other's back," people might look at you strangely. Yet if someone who had sex, even though it didn't feel right and left him with mixed feelings, answers: "Yeah, I got some," or "We got down really quick!" that person is the one who gets the attention in the locker room or during lunchtime gossip.

It seems that sex, no matter how unfulfilling, may be seen as a bigger deal in people's eyes than a truly intimate moment where everyone's clothes stay on. Here is another example of that: What do we call sexual behaviors (besides sex itself) such as kissing and touching? We call them foreplay. And what does foreplay mean? *Fore* means "before," so foreplay is "before play." And what would the "play" be in this case? The play is "sex." So if you think of all these things you can do with someone that are very close, pleasurable, and intimate as foreplay, they sort of lose their own meaning, even though kissing, touching, and simply spending time together can be very special to someone.

Batter Up! The Baseball Approach to Sex

Currently, many people think about sexual expression and activity using some form of the Baseball Approach to sex. In this way of thinking, the place where a couple starts their relationship is "sexual inexperience" and the end point or goal of the relationship is to have sex! By making sex the goal, it becomes the focal point of sexual expression, a couple's time together, and the relationship itself. Phrases like "Going all the way," and "Home run" come from this mind-set. Along the way to having sex, people progress along the bases in a specific order toward sex: getting to first base means kissing; second base means above-the-waist touching; third base, below-the-waist touching or oral sex. All of these sexual behaviors are seen as foreplay and therefore don't count as much as sex, the final goal. If you don't end up having sex, you end up "striking out."

There are some problems with thinking about sex as the goal of a relationship. First, it makes sex more of an accomplishment rather than a shared experience. Baseball is also a competitive game with winners and losers—not a way we want to think about sex. In baseball we think about statistics and ability, not a moment between two people. Sex is seen as a success, a victory, not a personal reason to be in a relationship if you follow the Baseball Approach.

Second, you can barely even know a person in order to reach the goal of sex; when you play baseball, you don't necessarily know who's on the other team.

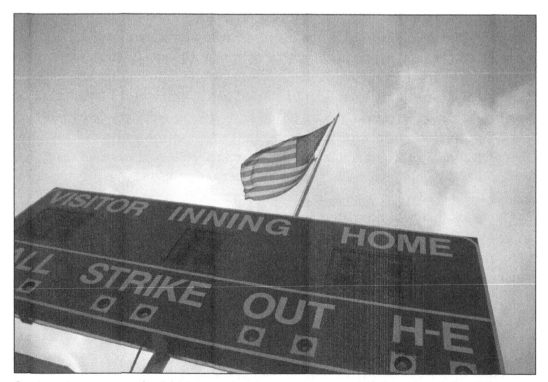

Sex is not a game, so don't keep score.

How wonderful, satisfying, or safe is it to have sex with someone who you do not know? Another thing, if people consider sex the goal of a relationship, they can go at it without really talking to each other about what they do and do not like—after all, we all know the rules of the game, right? Why do we need to discuss anything? In the Baseball Approach, partners are not encouraged to talk about their desires or comfort levels and may not find a good time to say when they are no longer feeling OK about what they are doing. This lack of communication can cause problems ranging from an unpleasant experience to more serious issues such as date rape.

Getting to Know Each Other: The Intimacy Approach to Sex

Instead of seeing sex from the Baseball Approach, sexual expression can be thought about using an approach that focuses on intimacy. Here, the priority of the relationship is not necessarily sexual—instead, the goal is to be intimate with another person. By making intimacy, and not sex, the goal of a relationship, you are not limiting the ways you can be with someone, but instead are opening the door to different forms of sexual expression and emotional expression. A relationship can become a lot more interesting, fun, and meaningful this way.

Placing intimacy as the goal of sexual expression emphasizes closeness for all involved and encourages communication between partners regardless of sexual experience. So in this way, if sex is a part of the relationship, both partners are more likely to enjoy the sexual experience since, as a part of intimacy, you are talking about your experiences and likes and dislikes together. This way of thinking about sexual expression encourages communication between sexual partners, because communication about thoughts, feelings, and who you are is a big part of being intimate with another person. Even though you might choose not to have sex in a relationship, there are many ways to be intimate with your partner that do not involve sexual behavior of any kind.

So why do I think the Intimacy Approach is better than the Baseball Approach to a relationship? First, the Intimacy Approach is the most flexible—there are so many ways to be intimate with another person. Some include sex and some do not. You can even choose not to have sex and have a great, intimate relationship with another. In fact, having sex isn't "all that" when thinking about intimacy, because you can certainly have sex with someone without being very close to that person. Expressing feelings, opening up to another, and sharing lives and experiences are the important activities and the focal point of couples who use the Intimacy Approach. So when you think of all the reasons why you want to be in a relationship, especially all the personal, not social, reasons you want to be in a relationship, I think you will find that the Intimacy Approach can make a lot of sense.

Hooray for Pizza!

Sexuality educator Al Vernacchio likes to think about having sex as ordering a pizza. When you order a pizza with someone else, you have to talk about what you want on it, much like you should talk about what sexual activities you do or do not want to do. Or you can even eat pizza by yourself (see the masturbation section). There are endless ways to eat a pizza and endless toppings. No one way is better than the other. The goal of eating pizza is to feel satisfied, which is a fine goal for a sexual encounter. Sometimes you want to feel stuffed, other times you just want a slice. Check out Vernacchio's TED Talk from 2012 to hear more.[b]

Masturbation: The Safest Sex of All

Of course there are times for everyone when a sexual partner is not available. During those times, some people choose to masturbate as a means of sexual release. Masturbation is the sexual issue that makes a lot of people uncomfortable. People will talk about sex, the importance of delaying sex, and how we need to improve sex education in schools. On television, shows will talk about affairs, "quickies," and many other sexual encounters. But who talks about masturbation? Not many, it seems. But there are a lot of myths and rumors about it. Like the one that says girls who masturbate are nymphomaniacs (girls who are addicted to sex). Boys, if you will, "get off" more easily; they have a bit more freedom to talk about masturbation, and it's more acceptable for them to admit doing it. But even then, there are limitations. There is the myth that boys who masturbate aren't getting any action in the real world, so they have to resort to pleasuring themselves. A similar myth is that boys who don't masturbate actually have a sex life, and that those who do masturbate do so because they don't have any "offers." Of course, these myths aren't true. People of all genders masturbate (and some people of all genders do not masturbate). People masturbate whether or not they have a partner, and their masturbation does not mean they are addicted to sex or have an unusually high sex drive.

Another thing that often goes along with masturbation is sexual fantasy. That is, as people masturbate it's common for them to think about certain sexual ideas or images to help them get aroused. Sexual fantasies are normal, and the types of

Masturbation in Song

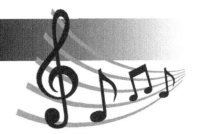

There are many songs that feature masturbation. Here are just a few:

- "I Touch Myself" by the Divinyls (1991)
- "Thinking about You" by Radiohead (1993)
- "Fingers" by Pink (2006)
- "B.O.B." by Macy Gray (2015)
- "Love Myself" by Hailee Steinfeld (2015)

---

fantasies people have are very different from one another. Also, having a sexual fantasy about something doesn't mean you want it to happen in real life. Fantasy is just that—fantasy, a time and place where you don't have to worry about the realities of a certain situation. It's a chance to let your mind wander to things that you think are sexy when you can control the outcomes in a safe, imaginary environment. So, try not to worry about what your sexual fantasies are, but at the same time, don't think that just because you imagine them while masturbating that they are things that you actually want to do with another person. They might be, but often they are not.

Masturbation—What It Is and Is Not

There are many good things about masturbation. Here are some of them:

1. It's 100 percent safe for people to do. By masturbating, you will not get pregnant, nor will you get an STD (and you will not go blind, sterile, or insane either).
2. People who masturbate know their bodies better. They can tell if there is something wrong "down there" because they are looking! And if you notice something wrong, you can go to a health-care provider to take care of it.
3. Knowing your body well also has another advantage—you know what does and does not work for you sexually. Knowing this can lead to better sexual communication between you and your current or future partner. Better communication is one of the most important factors in a healthy sex life.
4. Masturbating can make you more comfortable with your body. And being more comfortable with your body can make you more comfortable with yourself.

5. Masturbation helps people who choose to abstain from sexual intercourse for any reason. It's a good way to achieve sexual release because it can't hurt anyone, and it can help keep your impulses in check so you don't find yourself doing something you don't really want to do or aren't ready for.

Of course, nothing in life is 100 percent good. There are some downsides to masturbation as well:

- Some people who masturbate may feel guilty. They feel bad about it because they have been told by their parents or their religion that masturbation is wrong. People who feel guilty about masturbation need to think about the reasons they feel guilty and come to terms with their decisions. If they decide to continue masturbating, knowing that they may not always agree with their family or church and that that does not make them a bad person may help. If they decide not to masturbate, they can feel comfortable knowing they have the continued acceptance of the support systems in their life regarding that issue.
- There are a few people who masturbate too much. These people masturbate to the point where their schooling and social life suffer. This situation is very rare, but it does happen. There is no set amount of times one should or should not masturbate that is healthy. If you are able to continue to have a social life complete with outside activities and friendships, and your schoolwork is not suffering because of the time you are spending masturbating, you are not masturbating too much.

Question:

My penis has become "numb," I think from excessive masturbation. It is now harder for me to get sexually aroused and up to this summer I was masturbating at least once each day. How can I heal the "numbness"?
—Sixteen-year-old

Answer:

You really can't cause numbness from "excessive masturbation." "Excessive" really only has to do with the effect masturbation and the preoccupation with sex have on the other facets of your life (in other words, does it interfere with you developing social relationships or interfere with you getting your work done?). However, if you masturbate or have sex too frequently, it can make your urge to have sex less intense, and the sensations that you experience less pleasurable. If you masturbate less frequently, the sensations may improve.

Good Luck,

Dr. X, We Are Talking, teen health website

Historical Perspectives: The Jaded History of Masturbation

Today, health experts know that there are no harmful biological effects to masturbating. However, this was not the belief in the late 1700s and into the 1800s. In fact, back then, masturbation was referred to as "self-abuse" and "self-pollution" and was believed to result in long-term health problems, including insanity. Masturbation was considered especially dangerous for younger males (back then, doctors did not really believe that females masturbated at all!) because it would stunt their growth and make them unable to have children later in life. In 1886, John Harvey Kellogg (the inventor of Corn Flakes cereal), in his book on health, mentions that masturbation is "one of the most destructive evils ever practiced."[c]

It wasn't until the 1950s that health experts realized and admitted that masturbation had no bad health effects, but they still mainly considered it to be practiced by males only. Others back then did acknowledge that some females masturbated, but believed that if they did, it may "make more difficult the adjustments to the marriage partner"[d]—that is, if a girl masturbated before marriage, she might have trouble engaging in sex with her future husband.

Today, for the most part, health experts all finally agree that the only consequences of masturbation are psychological, resulting from possible guilt or anxiety if the person who is masturbating believes it's wrong according to his or her religion or parental beliefs. However, masturbation is hardly considered an acceptable topic for discussion. Take the more recent case of former surgeon general Dr. Joycelyn Elders. Elders was forced to resign in 1995 because of her controversial opinions on sex education, including her belief that masturbation is a healthy part of a young person's sexuality and therefore it should be taught in schools.

So, you might want to try masturbating, but are not sure how to go about it. Basically, masturbation is touching, rubbing, or otherwise stimulating your genitals (usually your penis or clitoris, but the sky's the limit: do whatever works for you. Try different things!) in ways that feel good to you. Although I am not going to tell you exactly how, here are some pointers to consider:

- Make sure you are in a private place where no one can disturb you. Lock doors if possible.
- Make yourself comfortable. It's important that you are in a physical place where you can be comfortable.
- Allow yourself to have whatever sexual fantasies you like. Fantasies are not bad, and do not necessarily reflect what you want to do in real life. Fantasies are what they are—thoughts in your head. Let them go.
- Use some lubricant to help your fingers. Your body will probably respond better to your touch if there is less friction. A water-based lubricant can help (saliva also works in a pinch).
- Do whatever feels good. There is no right or wrong way to masturbate. Experiment with different speeds and pressures; you know what works for you. The only "right" things to do are the things that feel good to you.
- It's OK if you do not masturbate to orgasm. For some it will take a few tries before you figure out how to orgasm through masturbation. Others may simply not care to reach orgasm—they just want to get aroused and then stop.

A final word: Learning about how your body works, discovering what your body does and does not like, and being in charge of your sexual desires are important skills to have. Masturbation can help with all of these things. But the most important thing to remember is only do what you feel comfortable doing. If masturbating is not for you, that's OK: you don't have to do it.

More about Joycelyn Elders

Dr. Joycelyn Elders was born in rural Arkansas in 1933, where she worked with her seven brothers and sisters in the fields. Always a top student, in 1960 she got her medical degree from the University of Arkansas (one of just three African American students to do so at the time). She then became chief pediatric resident. In 1987, Bill Clinton (then governor of Arkansas) named her director of the state's Department of Health. When Clinton became president, he named her surgeon general. She was forced to resign in 1995 (less than a year later) because of her controversial opinions about sex ed. Still a supporter of teen sex education, she is now a professor emerita at the University of Arkansas Medical Center.

SEXUALLY TRANSMITTED DISEASES

O ver six hundred thousand girls aged fifteen to nineteen get pregnant every year in the United States. Thinking about your own life and the people you know, it would not be surprising if you know someone who was pregnant before the age of twenty or who is now a young parent. Most young people know at least one person who has had this experience. However, do you know at least one person who has a sexually transmitted disease (an STD)? If you say no, you're not alone—not many young people think they know someone who has an STD. But guess what? More young people get an STD than get pregnant every year. In fact, half of sexually active people will get an STD by the time they are twenty-five years old, and one in four young people contract an STD every year.[1]

Why are there more cases of STDs than pregnancies every year? Here are a few reasons:

- Any body can get and carry an STD; only some bodies can get pregnant.
- Pregnancies can only happen during certain phases of the fertility cycle. Anyone can get an STD, no matter what time of the month.
- There are many ways to get an STD. There is only one way to get pregnant (we're not talking about artificial insemination here, folks).

Given all these facts, here's a question to ask yourself: Why is it that even though more young people get STDs than get pregnant, we know about the pregnancies in our school or social circle, but not the STD cases? Wouldn't it make sense that if there are three times as many STDs as pregnancies, we would know three times as many people with STD cases than with pregnancies? One would think, but there are reasons this is not the case:

- In public, you can tell if someone is pregnant after a few months. You cannot tell if people have an STD if you see them walking down the street.
- There are some people who talk about getting pregnant or getting someone pregnant. It's rarer to meet someone who discusses getting, or giving someone, an STD.
- People may turn to a friend if they are concerned about a pregnancy or possible pregnancy. People are less likely to turn to friends about concerns over STDs.
- Many people do not even know they have an STD when they do.

So, like an unexpected pregnancy, STDs are something young people (all people, for that matter) want to avoid when they have sex. But unlike pregnancy, which many young people eventually desire, an STD is not something anyone wants. Knowing the different types of STDs, what they look like, and how to avoid them is an important part of anyone's sex education.

STD Basics

As the name *sexually transmitted disease* suggests, a person can get an STD from having sex with a person who is already infected with the disease. However, having sex with someone is not the only way to get an STD. Some STDs can be transmitted by sharing needles (which can happen during IV drug use or while getting a tattoo using an unclean needle), and some STDs such as critters (or "pests") can be transmitted simply by sharing a towel with an infected person. However, sex is the main way STDs pass from one person to another. The trick is to realize that sex is not just a penis-in-vagina activity. Having anal sex or oral sex are also ways that STDs can be transmitted. In fact, herpes and gonorrhea are easily passed from one person to another through oral sex. Anal sex and oral sex are not safe behaviors when it comes to STD transmission. True, you cannot get someone pregnant those ways, but you (or someone else) can get infected.

There are three basic types of STDs: critters, bacteria, and viruses. Critters are just what they sound like—little pests that live on or just underneath your skin. They look like tiny, tiny bugs, and sometimes you can actually see them with your own eyes if you look closely enough. Although nasty sounding and unpleasant, critters can be the easiest and least invasive STDs to get rid of. All you have to do is wash yourself and all your belongings in really hot water using a special shampoo that you can get at your local pharmacist (read the label for specific directions). The two main types of critters are scabies and crabs. The bummer is that besides being easy to cure, they are relatively easy to catch. Although they are grouped under sexually transmitted diseases, you do not have to have sex with someone to actually get critters. Sharing a bed or a towel with someone who has scabies or crabs is enough to get them—all these critters have to do is crawl from one warm body to the next.

The next type of STDs is bacteria. The good thing about these STDs is that they can be cured—all you have to do is go to the doctor, take some antibiotics, and the disease is gone for good. The bad news is that these STDs often have no symptoms. You look fine, you feel fine, but you are not fine. It's only until months or years later that you realize something is wrong, and by then it may be too late to kill the STD with simple antibiotics. Long-term effects of untreated bacterial STDs include sterility (not being able to have children forever) and serious internal infections.

The last type of STD is the virus. Viral STDs unfortunately have no cure, but there are treatments. Like bacterial STDs, some viral STDs don't have any symptoms or don't have symptoms until they have progressed for a while.

Specific STDs: Recognize and React

Now that you know the basic categories of STDs, here are some descriptions of specific STDs that are pretty common among young people. If you see them on a partner, do not have sex with each other until that person gets checked out and cured or treated. If you see these symptoms on yourself, go to a doctor or health clinic as soon as you can to get the best possible treatment. Table 5.1 provides an overview of STDs by type.

Chlamydia

Type: Bacteria.
Symptoms: Over half of people with chlamydia have no symptoms. Those who do, experience a watery discharge, painful urination, itching, and burning.
Treatment: When diagnosed, chlamydia is easily treated and cured with antibiotics. It's important to take all of the medication prescribed to cure chlamydia, even if the symptoms or signs stop before all the medication is gone. It's possible to get this STD more than one time in your life.
If left untreated: Long-term effects include pelvic inflammatory disease (PID). Of those with PID, 20 percent will become infertile and 18 percent will experience intense, chronic, pelvic pain. If a woman with PID gets pregnant, she has a 9 percent chance of having a life-threatening tubal pregnancy (the fetus starts to grow in the fallopian tube—where there is no room for

it—instead of the uterus). Other people with untreated chlamydia can get a urethral infection (the urethra is the tube you pee out of). Testicles can become swollen and tender.

Fact: Seventy percent of all chlamydia cases are in young people under twenty-five.[2]

Gonorrhea

Type: Bacteria.

Symptoms: The early symptoms of gonorrhea are often mild if there are any at all (up to 80 percent have no symptoms at all). Even when there are symptoms, they can be so general that the gonorrhea is mistaken for a bladder or vaginal infection. The initial symptoms and signs include a painful or burning sensation when urinating and a vaginal or penile discharge that is yellow or bloody. Sometimes gonorrhea causes painful or swollen testicles. A person can also get gonorrhea in the anus (by having anal sex) or in the mouth (by having oral sex). Signs of an anal infection include discharge, anal itching, soreness, bleeding, and sometimes painful bowel movements. Infections in the throat cause few symptoms.

Treatment: When diagnosed, gonorrhea is easily treated and cured with antibiotics. It's important to take all of the medication prescribed to cure gonorrhea, even if the symptoms or signs stop before all the medication is gone. It's possible to get this STD more than one time in your life.

If left untreated: Untreated gonorrhea might result in pelvic inflammatory disease. Of those with PID, 20 percent will become infertile and 18 percent will experience intense, chronic, pelvic pain. If a woman with PID gets pregnant, she has a 9 percent chance of having a life-threatening tubal pregnancy. Gonorrhea can also cause epididymitis, a painful condition of the testicles that can lead to infertility. Gonorrhea can also infect the prostate and can lead to scarring inside the urethra, making urination difficult.

Hepatitis B

Type: Virus.

Symptoms: Many of the symptoms are general, like poor appetite, vomiting, and headaches. The more unique symptom is jaundice, which is the yellowing of the eyes and skin.

Treatment: There is a vaccine for hepatitis B—ask your doctor about it. Many people do eventually recover from hepatitis B; however, they are not completely cured.

Table 5.1. Which Are Which? STDs by Type

Bacteria (curable)	Critters (curable)	Viruses (not curable, but treatable)
Chlamydia	Pubic lice	Hepatitis B
Gonorrhea	Scabies	Herpes
Syphilis		HPV/genital warts
Trichomoniasis		HIV

If left untreated: You can recover, but some people suffer serious liver damage or cancer.

Herpes

Type: Virus.

Symptoms: Outbreaks of painful, bubbly blisters on the mouth, genitals, throat, and/or anus (depending on where point of contact was made). The sores then open up and ooze or bleed, then finally scab up and go away (they will come back again later). The entire genital area may feel very tender or painful. While transmission of herpes is most common during outbreaks, it can be spread from one person to another when there are no visible blisters.

Treatment: Herpes can never be completely cured, but staying healthy can help decrease outbreaks. Certain pills can also help make the symptoms less severe and outbreaks less common. There are also ways to make the sores less painful, such as keeping them clean and dry.

If left untreated: The outbreaks can become more severe and happen more often. These outbreaks are usually most noticeable within the first year following the first episode. But once you have herpes, you always have herpes, and transmission is possible. Talk to a health-care provider about being sexually active with herpes.

Question:

I kissed someone that had kissed someone else that might possibly have herpes in the mouth.

Can I get it?

—Eighteen-year-old

Answer:

Yes—it is possible. If you have ever had a cold sore in your entire life you may already have it. The Type 1 oral herpes virus is very common; most adults have already been infected in childhood. We recommend that people with active cold sores not kiss others, especially infants. Kissing a person who kissed a person is a bit far-fetched—but you can never say never with viral infections.

Sincerely,

Dr. X, We Are Talking, teen health website[3]

HIV/AIDS

Many people do not realize that HIV and AIDS are two different things. Even though they are closely related to each other, they are not the same and it is important to know the difference between them. To put it simply, HIV stands for human immunodeficiency virus. AIDS (acquired immune deficiency syndrome) is the end result of HIV infection. In other words, HIV is the virus that causes AIDS.

Here are the details about HIV:

Type: Virus.

Symptoms: You cannot rely on symptoms to tell if you have HIV. Many people who have HIV do not show symptoms of the disease for many years. The only way to tell if you have HIV is to get tested. In the same way, you cannot tell if a person has AIDS by looking for symptoms. The symptoms of AIDS are similar to the symptoms of many other diseases.

Treatment: There is no cure for HIV/AIDS. When someone tests HIV positive, that person should live a very healthy lifestyle to prolong life. There are many drugs that have been developed to help those with HIV/AIDS live longer and more comfortably.

If left untreated: AIDS is 100 percent fatal. Everyone who gets AIDS eventually dies from complications of the disease, even though there are some who have lived years after diagnosis.

Fact: One in five young adults believe there is a cure for AIDS or isn't sure if there is a cure.[4] It is important to remember that there is still no cure for AIDS, even if people are living longer with the disease thanks to advances in life-saving drugs.

HPV (Genital Warts)

Type: Virus.

Symptoms: Many types of HPV (human papillomavirus) have no symptoms. Some strains have genital warts that look like clusters of flesh-colored cauliflower bumps on your genitals. However, since these warts can pop up either inside or outside the body, they may be difficult to see. Genital warts are soft and usually itchy.

Treatment: Because genital warts are caused by a virus, they cannot be cured. However, there are chemicals that can burn them off of your body. Genital warts can also be frozen or cut off, or removed with a laser. However, there is a chance that they will come back again.

If left untreated: There is a link between HPV cancers of the cervix, vagina, anus, and penis. The good news is, there are vaccines on the market that prevent most kinds of HPV that cause cancer or warts. It is recommended that all young people get the HPV vaccine when they are twelve years old, or at least before they become sexually active.

HPV Vaccine

The HPV vaccine protects against four major types of HPV—two types that cause cancers and two types that cause genital warts. However, there are about forty types of HPV, so it's a good idea to get tested for all STDs and/or use condoms if you are sexually active in ways that can transmit STDs. Get the vaccine before your first sexual contact—it's been approved by the FDA to be given to young people ages nine through twenty-six—because that way it's guaranteed you haven't been exposed to the virus yet. But even if you have engaged in activities that could have exposed you to the virus, getting the vaccine is still a good idea because you can be protected against strains that you haven't come in contact with yet.

The vaccine is given in three doses. After the first dose, the second one is given two months later and the third dose six months after that. The shots can be a bit painful, but it's a lot better than getting genital warts or cancer.

Question:

I have not been sexually active for more than eighteen months, but the other day two small, red bumps appeared on the shaft of my penis. Could this just be a couple of pimples, or is there a chance that I could be showing symptoms of HPV even though I haven't had sex in over a year? Can I show the signs of genital warts this long after my last sexual encounter?

—Nineteen-year-old

Answer:

It is hard to tell what the bumps might be without seeing them. As you may know, the only real way of diagnosing genital warts is by visual inspection. Don't hesitate to see your doc if they do not go away or if you are curious about what they may be. The ones you describe could indeed be just pimple type lesions. But without seeing them, it's a guess. Yes, it is possible to not show any signs of several sexually transmitted diseases for months or years before they finally express themselves. Condom use is strongly recommended, as is care of selecting a partner. Genital warts or HPV, in particular, can be avoided nicely by using a condom.

Best,

Dr. X, We Are Talking, teen health website

Scabies and Pubic Lice

Type: Critters.

Symptoms: Extreme itching and redness in the genital area. You can sometimes see pubic lice, but scabies are too small to see without a microscope.

Treatment: Wash the body and all clothes, bedding, and so on, in a special insecticide soap that you can get at the pharmacy.

Movie Review: Dallas Buyer's Club (2013, 2h)

Set in 1985, at the start of the AIDS epidemic, a man who is diagnosed with HIV fights to get himself and others with the disease access to newly developed drugs. Matthew McConaughey won the Academy Award for Best Actor for playing the sick man who fights for his rights and those of others.

If left untreated: The critters will go to other parts of your body and the itching will get worse!

Syphilis

Type: Bacteria.

Symptoms: The symptom of the primary stage of syphilis is a single firm, round, small, and painless sore (called a chancre) on the genitals. The chancre will go away on its own in one to five weeks. However, even if the sore is gone, the syphilis is not. The second stage of syphilis starts when one or more areas of the skin break into a rash that usually does not itch. Sometimes the rashes are so faint they are not noticed. Rashes typically last two to six weeks and clear up on their own. If the syphilis still is not treated, it will eventually overtake the body, and can lead to brain deterioration, blindness, and liver failure years later. This last stage of syphilis is fatal (see "If left untreated").

Unethical Science

For forty years (1932–1972), the U.S. Public Health Service conducted experiments on almost four hundred African American men in Tuskegee, Alabama, who had syphilis. Although penicillin had been discovered, these men were not cured of their disease because doctors wanted to examine how late-stage syphilis affected black men as opposed to whites—the theory was that whereas whites died from neurological damage (i.e., they went mad), African Americans, who are more prone to heart disease, would die of heart failure. Because historical documents tell us how whites from syphilis died, experiments on whites were apparently not necessary. A journalist, Jean Heller, leaked the story in 1972, thus stopping the experiments. However, as a result of this experiment, twenty-eight men died of syphilis, one hundred died of related complications, forty wives had been infected, and nineteen children were born with the disease. It wasn't until 1997 that the government apologized for the Tuskegee experiments, when then-president Bill Clinton said, "The United States government did something that was wrong—deeply, profoundly, morally wrong."

Treatment: One dose of penicillin (an antibiotic) will cure a person who has had syphilis for less than a year. However, a person who has syphilis must not have sex with anyone until the sore is completely healed, or else the disease can be transmitted to a partner.

If left untreated: Syphilis can lead to brain deterioration, blindness, liver failure, and eventually death.

Trichomoniasis

Type: Parasite (it works like a bacteria).

Symptoms: Trichomoniasis causes a frothy, yellow-green discharge with a strong odor. The genital area will also itch and appear infected. The infection may cause discomfort during intercourse and urination. Some men may have irritation inside the penis, mild discharge, or slight burning after urination or ejaculation.

Treatment: Trichomoniasis can usually be cured with one dose of the prescription drug metronidazole.

If left untreated: The itching and burning may continue until trichomoniasis is treated.

If I Don't See It, I Don't Have It, Right?

Wrong!! It would be easy for people to believe that if they do not see or feel any of the symptoms of an STD, then they are STD-free. Unfortunately, this is not the case. If you read closely, you saw that some STDs rarely have any symptoms (chlamydia and gonorrhea are especially sneaky). That means, you could feel perfectly fine, yet you are actually infected with an STD. Knowing this, if you had to get an STD, would you rather:

1. Have no symptoms and feel great
2. Have symptoms—let it burn and itch

If you said "have no symptoms," I would like to try to convince you otherwise. The answer I prefer is "have symptoms." Sure, having symptoms is no fun, but symptoms can be a good thing. Having symptoms means you know you have the disease. Knowing you have the disease means that you know you need treatment. Knowing you need treatment means that you will hopefully get treatment. Getting treatment is not only good for you, but good for your partners (current and future) and the rest of society. Knowing you have an STD can help stop the spread of that STD. Make sense? When you get an STD, you want to have symptoms. Here's a story to help make this clearer:

Michael has sex with a person infected with gonorrhea. After a few days, he feels awful. It burns when he pees—so bad that it feels like razor blades. What does Michael do? Does he just continue through life as if nothing were wrong? Heck no! He is going to get checked to see what is going on! He wants to feel better. And when he does go to the clinic, he learns that he has gonorrhea. He gets some antibiotic pills and he is cured. He tells his partner to go in for testing, who then gets treated if necessary. This chain of gonorrhea is broken, thanks to symptoms and the actions of Michael and his partner.

Meanwhile, Monica has sex with a person infected with chlamydia. Like up to 80 percent of people, once she gets the disease, she has no symptoms. Monica feels healthy, despite the fact she's infected, and lives her life as if nothing is wrong. A few weeks later, she falls in love with a wonderful person at a party— they just seem to hit it off right away and they feel right together. They have sex, and she transmits the disease to her partner (not on purpose—she has no idea she has an STD). After six months together, they break up and start to date other people. Monica's ex is infected with chlamydia and also has no symptoms. That person also has sex with other people, transmitting the disease to another (who spreads the disease to others, and the chain continues). Meanwhile, Monica meets another great person, and after dating for five years, they decide to marry and have children. This young couple becomes frustrated after trying to have children for a year. A doctor's exam reveals that Monica is now infertile; her fallopian tubes are scarred due to the infections caused by the chlamydia she never knew she had.

The message of these two stories is, symptoms may stink in the short term, but when you look at the big picture, be thankful you were one of the lucky ones who was able to get treatment for an STD. Another message here is that if you have sex, get tested for STDs on a regular basis (like, once a year or even twice a year if you have unprotected sex or multiple partners). Get tested even if you feel fine. Get tested for your benefit and the benefit of others you kept from infection by breaking one of the chains of STD transmission.

Getting Tested for STDs

So, you think you might have an STD and you want to do something about it. Or, you have no idea if you have an STD and want to know for sure. Excellent! The next step is to get tested to see if you actually have an STD, and if so, what kind. There are basically three different types of tests that a doctor or health clinic will give you: a urine test, a blood test, or a swab test.

A urine test is when a health worker asks you to pee in a cup and then tests your urine for STDs; similarly, a blood test is when a health worker takes a sample of your blood (using a needle—it only stings for a second) and tests it. Finally, a swab test is when a health-care professional takes a sample of your cells from your vagina or the inside of your penis using a cotton swab (e.g., Q-tip). Then, a lab technician examines it under a microscope to determine the results.

All these tests take a few days to a week or two before there are results. Therefore, while you are waiting for the results of your test(s) do not have sex with anyone until you know if you are at risk for spreading a disease to someone else. Waiting is not everyone's favorite thing to do, but it's the right thing to do (see chapter 4 for more information on STD testing).

Choose the Right Health-Care Setting for You

Health-care providers such as doctors and nurses are great people to help you with STD testing and to discuss birth control options with. However, as you get older, the person you saw for your health concerns when you were a child may or may not be the best person for you. How can you tell if you've outgrown your childhood health-care provider? Consider the following:

- Does your health-care provider's waiting room have interesting magazines, or is it full of stuff that doesn't interest you?
- Does your health-care provider let you know that everything you say is confidential, unless it is a threat to your life?
- Does your health-care provider allow the two of you privacy during your visit, or is a parent with you all the time?
- Does your health-care provider ask questions about sex, alcohol, drugs, and/or your diet? (When doctors ask questions, it is not because they are nosy, but because they care about your health!)
- Will your health-care provider arrange for a separate, private billing if you wish to set up a private visit between the two of you?

A young person has a right to make a confidential visit to the doctor's office—in fact, it is your right to get tested for pregnancy and/or STDs, or ask about drug use, without your parent's knowledge.

If you feel you have "outgrown" your health-care provider, talk to a parent about it. Your parent can call your health plan to see if there is anyone in the health plan who specializes in adolescents and/or young adults, not just kids. To find a health-care provider who specializes in the health of people your age, go to the Society for Adolescent Medicine at www.adolescenthealth.org. You also

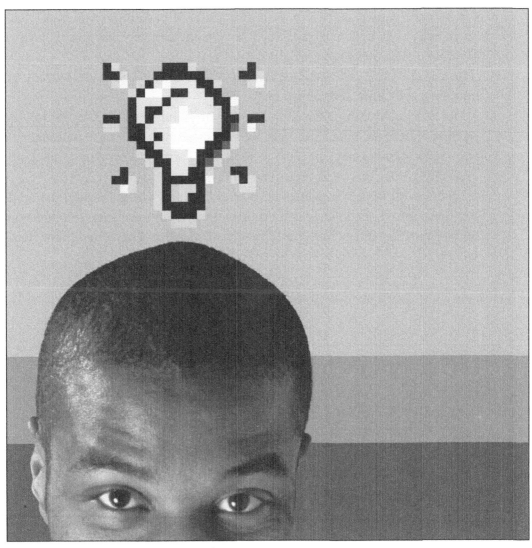

Getting tested for STDs is a good idea.

can drop by a health clinic or a school-based health center to get information on STDs, birth control, or any other questions about your sexual health.

Talking to Your Partner

If you are diagnosed with an STD, you absolutely must tell your partner or partners about it. Look at it this way: if someone you were sexual with had an STD, you would want that person to tell you so you could get treated. Telling someone you might have exposed him or her to a health problem and as a result both of you might be spreading it to other people is the right thing to do. There are a few different ways you can tell someone about the STD:

- Find a quiet time to talk. Say something like "I care about you and I want to do what I believe is right. So, I have something to tell you. I have an STD, and that means you might have it too."
- The clinic where you were tested for STDs might call your partner for you. Ask the clinic about its policy.
- Write a note explaining the situation if you honestly can't face up to your partner. There are some apps and websites that will break the news for you (but some cost money; be sure to read the Terms of Service of each one carefully before disclosing sensitive information).
- If you are no longer in touch with your partner, write that person a letter. Send a text. Find that person. You are helping not just you and your former partner, but possibly others as well. Be proud of yourself for doing what's right to help prevent the spread of an STD.

Staying safe makes sex more enjoyable for all.

CONTRACEPTIVES

··

There are a lot of ways to try to prevent yourself from being involved in a pregnancy. In order to make it easier for you to choose the right method, the birth control options in this chapter are broken down into four different categories: (1) timing; (2) using a barrier; (3) using artificial hormones; (4) having surgery (I won't cover this last type of option, because it's generally not available for young people). Some ways are more effective than others. Some ways help prevent not only pregnancy but also sexually transmitted diseases (STDs). Reading about all the different methods can help you decide which is right for you.

A friendly reminder: Preventing pregnancy and preventing STDs are not always the same thing. While there are many ways to prevent pregnancy and a few ways to prevent the STDs that you read about in chapter 5, there are only two things you can do to reduce your chances of both getting STDs and experiencing an unwanted pregnancy. Those two ways are

1. Choosing not to have sex (see chapter 3)
2. Using a condom

Because these two options take care of both getting an STD and having an unplanned pregnancy, they are talked about more in depth than the others. Getting rid of two concerns with one action is pretty efficient, so choosing not to have sex or using a condom if you decide to have sex are pretty good choices in my book.

As you read through all these birth control options, think about which one might be best for you, whether you are currently having vaginal intercourse or think you might have it someday in the relatively near future. Here are some things to consider while reading about all these options:

- *Effectiveness:* How well does it work when you use it perfectly every single time? How well does it work if you don't always use it correctly?
- *Cost:* How much do you need to pay up front? How much do you need to pay to maintain the method?

- *Access:* Some methods require a trip to the doctor, while others just require a trip to the nearest drugstore. Which option is better for you?
- *Side effects:* Do you have any health concerns that might prevent you from using a particular method?
- *How often you need to think about it:* Some methods you need to think about every day, or every time you have sex. Other methods are good for months or even years. Are you the type who is good at remembering things, or do you prefer not to think about something all the time?
- *Partner involvement:* No matter who is actually using the birth control method, both partners need to be supportive of each other in order to increase the chances it is used consistently and correctly. What does your partner prefer when it comes to contraceptives? If your partner doesn't want to use anything, then that person may not be the best for you.
- *Your sexual habits:* Are you in a monogamous relationship? How spontaneous are you when it comes to sex? Different methods are better for different sexual styles.

If after reading this chapter you are still not sure which contraceptive method is best for you, there are online tools at Bedsider.org and SexualityandU.ca that take you through a series of questions to help you decide. Talking to a health-care provider is also an excellent option. Choosing a way to reduce your chances of an unplanned pregnancy is important. Use all the resources you have to help you decide which option is best for you and your lifestyle.

Timing Methods

One way to prevent a pregnancy from happening is not to have sex when both parties are fertile. We know, thanks to chapter 1 or knowledge you had before, that the only way to cause pregnancy is for a sperm to fertilize an egg that is mature and ready. And although modern science has created many ways for this to happen, the only way this fertilization happens that concerns us is by having vaginal intercourse during ovulation. So, how can we prepare ourselves and reduce the chances of being involved in an unplanned pregnancy? There are three ways to do it without using contraception, which rely on the timing of sexual activity: leaving it to chance, using the withdrawal method, and using the rhythm method. These methods tend not to work very well, as you will find out, and they all take hard work. Still, I present them so you have a complete picture of all your options. Decide for yourself and your partner which are good options, and which ones are not right for you.

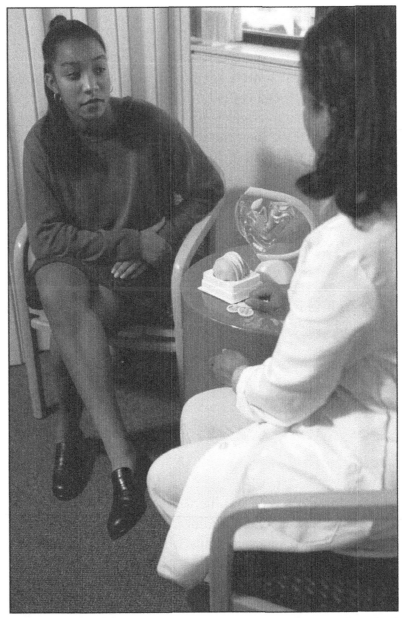

Health-care providers can help guide you to a birth control method that's right for you.

Fact

Forty percent of teens who are having vaginal sex with their partners say that they use contraception every time they have sex. That means a lot of people are not being as safe as they could be![a]

Leave It to Chance

One way to try not to get pregnant is to have sex and just hope. This is the most ineffective method of birth control around. In fact, out of one hundred couples who just leave it to chance, eighty-five will experience a pregnancy after just one year. That is more than eight couples out of ten. That is a lot. Simply put, luck and hope do not work in the long run. Sure, it may work one time, maybe even two or three. But make this a habit, and a pregnancy is highly likely.

Leaving It to Chance Summary

> *How it works:* It doesn't.
> *What makes it a good choice:* Nothing at all.
> *Why it might not be right for you:* You are smarter than that.
> *How to get it:* There is nothing to "get" in order to use this method, but then again, it's not really a contraceptive method at all.
> *Cost:* There are a lot of costs associated with leaving things to chance—stress, a high risk of pregnancy, and the costs of dealing with an unplanned pregnancy, to name just a few.
> *Wait time until it works:* It doesn't work. Don't choose this option, please.

Withdrawal

Withdrawal is a commonly used but ineffective way for people to prevent pregnancy. It happens when the penis is removed from the vagina before ejaculation. The problem is, there are many reasons why this method can go wrong very quickly. First, the guy has to be in total control of ejaculation and that's difficult to do: ejaculation can sneak up on a guy sooner than he thinks and the "pull out" will not happen in time. Second, tiny drops of pre-ejaculate, or pre-cum, come out of the penis before ejaculation (see chapter 1). This pre-cum sometimes has sperm and STD germs in it, so it is possible that a partner can still get pregnant or infected even before ejaculation. Finally, sometimes it's not easy to stop; the sex feels good and the couple, or one person, could change their minds about pulling out and end up having unprotected sex.

Withdrawal Summary

> *How it works:* The penis is removed before ejaculation.
> *What makes it a good choice:* It's better than nothing—barely.

Why it might not be right for you: There are many better options.

How to get it: There's nothing to get in order to use this method, but it's not worth the risk.

Cost: Free, but it's a big gamble.

Wait time until it works: Forever.

How well does it work: It fails over 20 percent of the time in young people.

What can go wrong: Ejaculation can happen sooner than expected, and pre-cum carrying infections and sperm can lead to an STD or pregnancy.

Natural Family Planning

The concept behind natural family planning is that a couple pays attention to the signals of the uterus and cervix and other parts of the body enough to know when ovulation is likely to happen (or is happening). The theory goes that if partners know when ovulation will happen, then they know when fertilization can and can't happen, and thus they know when to have sex in order to have or avoid having a baby.

However, like most theories, this one has its loopholes. And, like all contraceptive methods, this one has a failure rate—one that is particularly high for young people. This is because natural family planning requires a regular menstrual cycle that is very predictable and very dependable. For the most part, young women simply do not have regular menstrual cycles. There is too much growing, stress, and newness to the whole thing for it to be really settled. Plus, in order to really understand the natural family planning method and to really get to know her cycle inside and out, a woman should go to a class (through a church, health clinic, or hospital) for up to two years. That is a long time and a lot of dedication in order to avoid a pregnancy. Thus, natural family planning is not a recommended form of birth control for younger people, in the eyes of health-care professionals.

Natural Family Planning Summary

How it works: Cervical mucus, body temperature, and menstrual calendars are checked to try to figure out when ovulation may occur.

What makes it a good choice: Women using this method get to know their bodies very well. There are some religions that only accept this form of birth control.

Why it might not be right for you: It's a very unreliable method for young people because of teens' unpredictable menstrual cycles, it takes a long time to learn, and there is no protection against STDs.

How to get it: Take a class and read a lot in order to understand how it works.

Cost: Classes vary in price.

Wait time until it works: It takes two years to learn, to be extra safe.

How well does it work: It fails 24 percent of the time.

What can go wrong: The menstrual cycle is irregular and ovulation might happen when it's unexpected. Sperm can live up to six days after ejaculation, thus "hanging" around until ovulation, making fertilization possible.

Barriers: Keeping Sperm and Ova Away from Each Other

Barrier methods of birth control work by preventing sperm from getting near the egg. No contact between the sperm and the egg equals no pregnancy. The cool thing about these methods is that they can also help prevent the spread of STDs the same way they prevent pregnancy—by preventing the transmission of fluids from person to person. A "wall" does it all. Barrier methods are used at or near the time people are having sex. They do not remain on or inside the body the way hormonal methods do. If you are a person who does not have sex all that often but wants to be prepared, a barrier method might be the right choice for you.

Condoms

There are two types of condoms—those designed to go on penises and those designed to be inserted into a vagina. Here, we are going to focus on those that are used on penises because they are much more common, cheaper, and easier to access. For more information on female condoms, visit www.bedsider.org. Condoms have been used by millions of couples for over a century for the purpose of preventing pregnancies and the spread of STDs. Condoms are made from a variety of materials. Most condoms are made of latex. Latex is a type of rubber that is also used to make surgical gloves and other protective barriers. These condoms are the cheapest ones, but sometimes allergies make them not a good choice for some people. The good news is that there are condoms made of other materials—polyurethane, polyisoprene, and lambskin. Condoms made of these materials are sometimes harder to find and they are often more expensive, but they are reported by some to feel better and increase pleasure (this is especially true for those made of polyisoprene).

Condoms are good to use during sex because they protect against both pregnancy and STDs. An important exception to this is lambskin condoms—those may not be effective in preventing STDs, so be careful using those. You can use

History of Condoms

Condoms have been around for quite some time. There are cave paintings of condoms in France. The ancient Egyptians used condoms made of linen around 1000 BC. These linen condoms were tested in the 1500s in Italy; it was found that those people who used them did not get syphilis. Thus, it was officially proven that condoms helped prevent the spread of STDs. The latex condoms of today were first available in the 1880s, although they were not commonly used until the 1930s. Today, billions of condoms are manufactured worldwide every year. For a more complete history, check out http://www.avert .org/condoms.htm.

condoms for all kinds of sex: oral, anal, and vaginal. Also, condoms are pretty cheap and you can get them without a prescription. In this section, we are going to take an extra close look at condoms, how they work, and how to use them effectively. We are going to give this form of birth control the most attention because it's one of the three methods of safer sex, along with choosing not to have sex and testing plus monogamy.

Where Can You Get Condoms?

Condoms are the easiest and cheapest birth control method to get (besides choosing not to have sex). You can get condoms at health or family planning clinics, drugstores, grocery stores, the doctor's office, convenience stores, special condom stores, and even in vending machines. Sometimes condoms are only available behind locked cabinets in stores. This is because some store chains and owners believe that condoms should not be easily accessible to everyone and want these items in a more controlled environment; others lock them away because they are more likely to be stolen than other items. Having condoms locked away can sometimes make them difficult to buy, because you have to ask someone who works at the store to get them. While this can feel embarrassing or challenging, I hope you feel proud asking for them, because it shows that you are being responsible and respectful toward yourself and your partner.

Lubricant: The Condom's Best Friend

It's possible—very likely, even—that you have heard of condoms before picking up this book. Even if you have never seen one or used one, condoms are advertised in magazines and on the radio. They are talked about in public service announcements concerning the prevention of AIDS. You can see them in stores and at a clinic office, or at a friend's house. However, it's rare that people talk about lubricants, which are an important part of condom use.

Lubricants designed for sex are water-based substances that reduce friction. Reducing some friction during sex can be a good thing because it can prevent the condom from tearing, and it can make sex more comfortable and pleasurable. If you are using a latex condom, sexual lubricants need to be water-based because other types of lubricants—those that are oil-based—actually eat away at latex and make holes in condoms. Some examples of oil-based lubricants are most lotions, Vaseline, and cooking oil. You can find water-based lubricants where condoms are sold. Common brand names of water-based lubricants include Wett, Astroglide, and KY Jelly. The good news is if you use non-latex condoms, then it is OK to use oil-based lubricants.

How to Be a Condom-Savvy Person

Before using a condom, look at the condom still in its wrapper. It should have an expiration date on it. Make sure the condom you use is not expired. Expired condoms are more likely to tear or may already have a hole in them. Just as you would not drink expired milk, you should not use expired condoms. Store your condoms properly. Condoms need to be kept in a cool, dry place when not in use. They should not be kept in a car, where the heat can get really intense, or in a pants pocket, where they can get crumpled up and also hot, being close to your body. Storing condoms in a backpack or purse can be a good idea, if they are kept in their own pocket and aren't junked in with the rest of your stuff. Jacket pockets and front shirt pockets are okay places to put condoms for convenient access. Just keep them out of your pants pockets where the condom can get too close to the body.

Putting on a Condom: Dos and Don'ts for the Safest and Best Time Possible

Now, the moment has come for sex, and you are ready to put on the condom. How do you do it? It's easy, once you get the hang of it, but practicing does help. Your two fingers are a great prop to use in order to practice using a condom before you need to use one with a partner. Read on to learn some great pointers on the process.

Step 1: Open the Package

First, make sure that the penis is hard before you put on the condom. Condoms do not stay on unless the penis is hard. Push the condom to one side of the package and carefully tear the opposite corner. No teeth, no ripping with abandon, as you do not want to tear the condom.

Step 2: Determine Upside Down versus Right Side Up

Before you unroll the condom, take a second to look at it. There is a right way and a wrong way to unroll the condom. Check out the picture to see what I mean. Unrolling the condom the wrong way will increase the chance of tearing it, so take that extra moment to make sure you are doing it right. This may be difficult to do when it's dark, so either turn on the lights to put on a condom, or become familiar with condoms to get a good feel for them and know the difference between right side up and upside down.

Step 3: Get Out the Lubricant

Next, put a few drops—three or four is plenty—of lube on the inside of the condom (don't overdo it here; things could get too slippery and messy). You want to

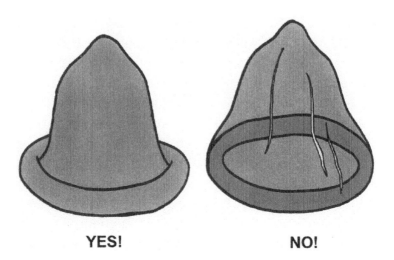

YES!   NO!

There is a right way and a wrong way to put on a condom. *Image by Amy Nelson* put lube inside the condom because it reduces the chance of the condom breaking. Also, the lubricant increases pleasure for the person wearing the condom because lubrication actually helps transmit the heat of sex through the latex of the condom.

Step 4: Put It On

Now you know the right direction the condom goes on the penis and you have put a few drops of lube inside. You are ready to put it on. With one hand, pinch the tip of the condom (that little nub at the top) to leave room at the tip. Why do you want to do this? To leave room for the semen/cum/ejaculate. You also want to leave room at the tip of the condom so that it's more comfortable for the person wearing it.

Then, with other hand, form an "OK" sign, and roll the condom down all the way to the base of the penis, while still pinching the tip of the condom. The OK method decreases the chances of tearing the condom with fingernails. Once the condom is on, the condom will have lots of room at the tip for the semen, but the rest of it is on snugly so that it will not fall off. Next, you can put lubricant on the outside of the condom for your partner's pleasure (if your partner wants it, that is) and to help prevent the condom from tearing.

Finally, please note that taking off the condom properly is just as important as putting it on properly, so thus continues the lesson.

Step 5: Take It Off

There are two things to remember about taking off the condom: First, do it right after ejaculation, because after that the penis starts to get limp, the condom will no longer stay on, and you don't want to spill anything inside your partner. Second, you want to grab the base of the condom and pull it off. If the guy simply pulls out without holding on to the condom, the condom can stay inside his partner and spill semen. The whole point of wearing the condom is foiled! Finally, tie the condom like a balloon so nothing spills out of it and throw it away. Do not flush the condom down the toilet as condoms can clog toilets (and possibly leave you with either a large plumbing bill or at least an unromantic encounter with a plunger).

One final thing before I declare you a condom expert: condoms can be used once and only once. As soon as the erection is lost or ejaculation happens (or both), that condom cannot be used again! Once a condom is used, you should throw it away properly, as just described. If you want to have sex again, you must get a new condom.

You now know how to put a condom on properly and take it off successfully so that it can be an effective way to prevent pregnancy and STDs. Congratulations! It's a good idea to practice putting condoms on by using your fingers, an appropriately shaped fruit or vegetable, or even yourself if that's an option (please note that food options, while good for practice, are not representative of the actual size of your average penis—fruits and vegetables tend to be a lot bigger). Practicing putting a condom on makes things easier when it's time to get it right and increases your sense of confidence that you are practicing safer sex so you can better enjoy the moment with your partner. Also, practicing putting on a condom when you are by yourself, in a quiet and calm environment, will make things go smoother when you are with a partner and possibly a little nervous and/or excited. Finally, your confidence can look pretty darn sexy if you know what you're doing next time you are with someone. So many reasons to practice!

Avoid Breakage!

If condoms have to undergo all these quality control tests, why do so many people hear and have their own stories about condoms breaking? For the most part, the reason condoms break is not because they are faulty or made wrong, but because of human error. The people using the condoms do things that make breakage more likely. Here are the most common reasons condoms break:

1. There was not enough room at the tip of the condom. When you roll a condom onto the penis, be sure to leave some room at the top. This is so that when the guy ejaculates, there is a place for the semen to go! If you stretch the condom tightly over the head of the penis, this will not only be uncomfortable, but also increase the chances of it breaking.
2. The condom was not stored properly. If the condom is near heat (in someone's back pocket, in the glove compartment of a car), the material weakens, which makes it more likely that it will break. Condoms need to be kept in a cool (not cold) place. A nightstand, in a purse, or in a coat pocket are good places. Just make sure they stay away from sharp objects!
3. A fingernail tears the condom while it's being put on. File those nails and be careful! And no ripping open the condom package with your teeth. You could rip the condom that way, too.
4. The wrong type of lubricant was used. Remember, only water-based lubricants should be used if you choose a latex condom. Oil-based lubricants such as lotions, Vaseline, and massage oils should not be used on condoms made of latex (they are OK for other kinds of condoms).

By taking these condom-breaking reasons into consideration the next time you have safer sex, you will be having even safer "safer sex"!

Which Condom Should I Use?

You have decided to have sex and have talked to your partner about protection. The two of you have decided to use a condom to protect yourselves against STDs and/or pregnancy. Congratulations! That is a good step toward practicing safer sex. But then you ask—what condoms should you use? I've already talked about the fact that there are different types of condoms based on the material they are made of. There are also many brands of condoms—Lifestyles, Trojan, Kimono, Beyond 7, Maxx, just to name a few. All condoms pass very strict quality control tests before they are allowed to be sold in the United States. If you buy a condom in the United States, no matter what country it was made in, you can be assured that it has been tested for strength, durability, and everything else you might be concerned about. Here are some other things to consider when deciding what condoms to choose.

Size can matter, so choose the right condom for you. There are condoms that are snug fitting, condoms that are regular sized, and condoms that have extra room either all over or just at the top, or "head." If you have trouble ejaculating too soon, you might want to try a snugger fitting condom. These condoms say "snugger fit" on them, and most condoms made in Japan tend to have a snugger fit.

Most people will want to get an average-sized condom. If you're not sure which kind to get, first try a condom that does not say it's snug or has extra room. Then, once you try it out, you can go from there. Yes, there are condoms that are bigger out there. But bigger is not always better. Unless you are really, truly, honestly someone who needs a bigger condom, I would not suggest getting one. A bigger condom can be baggy on some, and that will cause it to feel bulkier and it might interfere with pleasure. However, some people like the bagginess because they like the friction that goes along with it.

Next, when it comes to feel, thinner might be better. Because all condoms have already passed strength tests, you can rest assured that any condom you buy will be strong enough, no matter how thin it feels. In general, condoms that are made of polyurethane tend to be thinner and better at transferring heat. This means it may feel more "natural." Japanese condoms as a general rule are thinner than those made in America. Trojans have a reputation of being thicker and rubberier than most condoms.

You may also notice that condoms come in many different colors and textures. These features are mostly for fun. Certainly color does not affect the condom itself, but it can make sex more entertaining and interesting. Some people, though, appreciate textures: ribs, bumps, and other textures can add pleasure for some, while others do not notice the difference. The only way to know if you like them is to try them out yourself.

A word of warning, however: Watch out for condoms that say they are "novelty." These condoms do not protect you. These condoms are often found in bathroom vending machines at rest stops, clubs, and gas stations. Why they even make novelty condoms, I do not know. I personally think they are misleading and irresponsible on the part of manufacturers. People go out of their way to be protected, be responsible, by buying a condom, only to discover the condom used does not protect against STDs or an unplanned pregnancy. It's simply not fair to have to read the fine print in these situations. One of the novelty condom culprits is the glow-in-the-dark condom. Most of these are totally useless when it comes to protecting yourself (unless all you need to do is find your partner's penis when the lights are off). With so many other fun options, it's best to try another kind.

Question:

My boyfriend and I are getting really close. We have been talking about sex and we both agreed we would never have sex without a condom. However, neither of us knows what size condoms come in and how sizing works. Could you help us?

—Sixteen-year-old

Answer:

All condoms are not the same. Condoms come in different thicknesses, with different shapes (i.e., the same width from top to bottom, smaller at the bottom, contoured, reservoir tip, etc.), ribbed or dotted (inside or out), lubricated or nonlubricated, and in different colors. Only you can decide what is pleasurable for you. I would encourage you to try different condoms until you find the one you like the best. Many people like the micro-thin condoms for enhanced sensation, and you may like condoms that have ribbing or dots on the inside, which also enhance sensation.

An important thing about using condoms is to remember to use adequate lubrication to decrease friction and enhance pleasure. You can use a drop or two of water-based lubricant (like KY Jelly, Millennium, Probe, etc.) on the inside of the condom to enhance your pleasure, and a drop or two outside the condom to increase your partner's pleasure and reduce friction.

Good for you for thinking about this!

Dr. X, We Are Talking, teen health website[b]

Condom Summary

How it works: The semen gets trapped inside the condom, preventing semen and possible STDs from entering another person. The condom protects the person wearing it from potential STDs by acting as a coat or shield.

What makes it a good choice: It's cheap, easy to get a hold of, and pretty effective.

Why it might not be right for you: You or your partner may be allergic to the latex.

How to get them: Pretty much any drugstore, convenience store, or grocery store will have them.

Cost: They are anywhere from free to ten dollars for a box of twelve.

Wait time until it works: As soon as the penis is erect, put it on and you are ready to go.

How well does it work: Condoms have a failure rate of only 2 percent after a year of sex—as long as they are used consistently and correctly. If they are not used properly, 18 percent of couples will get pregnant if they use condoms after a year of sex.

What can go wrong: A condom can break or slip off. A guy might take the condom off improperly and spill semen into his partner. But by reading this section you found out how to avoid these problems as best as you can!

The Sponge

The sponge is a small, round piece of foam (about two inches around) with a piece of thick, soft string attached to it. It is inserted into the vagina so that the cervix is blocked, preventing sperm from fertilizing an egg. It also contains spermicide as extra protection from an unplanned pregnancy. You can buy sponges either online or in some stores. Sponges work for about twenty-four hours after they are inserted, so a couple can have vaginal intercourse multiple times during those hours without needing to change the sponge. However, you need to leave a sponge in your body for at least six hours after ejaculation to make sure the sperm do not survive and sneak by once you remove it!

Sponge Summary

How it works: It serves as a barrier close to the cervix to prevent sperm from getting through to the egg. It also releases spermicide for added protection.

What makes it a good choice: It's easy to use. It doesn't require a visit to a health-care professional.

Why it might not be right for you: You may not feel comfortable reaching inside your body to put the sponge in. It may not fit well.

How to get it: You can buy it online or in some stores.

Cost: Sponges are around fifteen dollars for three.

Wait time until it works: It works right away—just make sure it's in snugly!

How well does it work: The typical use failure rate is 12 percent in people who have never been pregnant.

What can go wrong: It can slip or not be put in correctly in the first place.

Diaphragm/Cervical Cap

The diaphragm and the cervical cap are both dome-shaped pieces of latex that fit inside the vagina to cover the cervix. This way, these methods act as barriers to prevent sperm from getting near the egg so fertilization will not take place. The diaphragm is a larger device, while the cervical cap is designed to fit more snugly, so it's smaller. Both of these birth control devices need to be prescribed by a doctor. They come in different sizes, and a woman needs to be fitted to see which one is best for her. In order for these methods to work most effectively, spermicide should be used with both to add extra protection from unwanted pregnancies. Note: You need to leave either of these devices in your body for at least six hours after ejaculation to make sure the sperm do not survive and sneak in after vaginal intercourse! You can use them more than once during a sexual encounter, but new spermicide needs to be applied each time for them to be as effective as possible.

Diaphragm Summary

How it works: It provides a barrier and holds spermicide close to the cervix to prevent sperm from getting through to the egg.

What makes it a good choice: It's easy to use.

Why it might not be right for you: You may not feel comfortable reaching inside your body to put the diaphragm in. It may not fit well.

How to get it: Your doctor helps find the right size and writes a prescription for it.

Cost: The diaphragm is around twenty dollars, plus the cost of the fitting at the clinic or doctor (which can be expensive). The spermicide is less than ten dollars a tube and is good for several applications.

Wait time until it works: Some health-care professionals suggest using a backup method for the first few times to make sure it fits OK and does not fall out. It works right away, once you get the hang of putting it in, and can be put in six hours before vaginal intercourse.

How well does it work: It fails between 6 and 12 percent of the time.

What can go wrong: It can slip or not be put in correctly in the first place.

Cervical Cap Summary

How it works: It fits snugly over the cervix to prevent sperm from getting through to the egg. Spermicide also helps kill sperm.

What makes it a good choice: It's easy to use.

Why it might not be right for you: You may not feel comfortable reaching inside your body to put the cervical cap in. It may not fit well.

How to get it: Your doctor helps find the right size and writes a prescription for it.

Cost: The cervical cap can cost up to sixty dollars, plus the cost of the clinic or doctor visit (which can be expensive). The spermicide is less than ten dollars a tube and is good for several applications.

Wait time until it works: Some health-care professionals suggest using a backup method for the first few times to make sure it fits OK and does not fall out. It works right away, once you get the hang of putting it in, and can be put in twenty-four hours in advance of having sex.

How well does it work: It's over 90 percent effective, with spermicide. It's less effective if spermicide is not used.

What can go wrong: It can slip or not be put in correctly in the first place.

Spermicide

Spermicide works because it stops sperm from moving. It comes in many different forms: jelly, foam, and little suppositories (pill-like things that are inserted into the vagina). Although it can be used alone as birth control, spermicide is usually used with a barrier such as a condom, diaphragm, or cervical cap in order to be most effective. Therefore, for the best protection, use spermicide with a diaphragm, cervical cap, or even a condom for more protection against both an unplanned pregnancy and STDs. And if you know you are more protected, you will be able to relax and enjoy the moment more. Preparing in advance for sex means being able to worry less about possible unwanted consequences.

Spermicide Summary

How it works: It prevents sperm from moving and getting to the egg.

What makes it a good choice: It's easy to use and is available in the drugstore.

Why it might not be right for you: It's not the most effective birth control method out there. It can get a little messy.

How to get it: Buy it at your local drugstore or online.

Cost: Spermicide is anywhere from five to ten dollars, depending on the type, where you get it, and how much you're getting.

Wait time until it works: It depends on the type you use. Some work right away, like the foam and jelly, while suppositories take about half an hour to expand to their full form.

How well does it work: It fails 18 percent of the time if used consistently and correctly. Typically, the failure rate is 28 percent.

What can go wrong: Not enough spermicide is used, the couple does not wait long enough for the spermicide to work, or some sperm simply get by. It's best to use spermicide with a diaphragm or cervical cap.

Question:
What happens to spermicide after sex?
—Twenty-year-old in Wisconsin

Answer:
After spermicide is inserted into the vagina, it gradually oozes out over the next day or so. It is not absorbed into the body.
Dr. X, We Are Talking, teen health website

Hormonal Methods

Hormonal methods work by preventing ovulation—some "trick" the body into believing it's pregnant; others simply prevent an egg from implanting or being released/maturing in the first place. Hormonal methods remain inside the body at all times—they are not just used when engaging in sexual intercourse. They do not prevent the spread of STDs. Therefore, hormonal methods are best used by people who are having sex often with only one faithful partner. Also, both members of the couple need to be STD-free, or they may infect and reinfect one another until they get treatment. If STDs are a concern, condoms can also be used.

Intrauterine Device (IUD)

IUD is a small T-shaped device that is placed all the way into the uterus by a health-care professional. While the person with an IUD cannot feel it in there, there is a little wiry string that hangs outside the uterus and in the vagina so that the user can make sure that the IUD is still in place (a partner can sometimes feel the strings with a penis or fingers). There are two kinds of IUDs. One has a band of copper around it and can stay inside the body for up to twelve years. The other type has a small amount of the hormone progestin. There are three different kinds of IUDs with progesterone, each slightly different in size, hormonal dose, and length of time it can stay in the body (between three and six years). Not that long ago, it was thought that IUDs were not a good option for young people, especially those who had never been pregnant before. This is no longer the case! IUDs are a great option for young people who do not wish to become pregnant for a long time. They are over 99 percent effective, involve little fuss, and last for years.

IUD Summary

How it works: It works by preventing sperm from fertilizing eggs.

What makes it a good choice: Once it's in you, it does its job without you having to pay much attention to it.

Why it might not be right for you: You might not like the idea of having a small device inside of you. An IUD provides no protection against STDs.

How to get it: A doctor would put it in for you.

Cost: IUDs can cost up to $350, including the doctor visit.

Wait time until it works: It works immediately.

How well does it work: Very! It's one of the most effective contraceptive methods around.

What can go wrong: The IUD may not remain in place, making the user at risk for pregnancy. The user can get pelvic inflammatory disease.

Birth Control Pills

Birth control pills, or "the pill," are the most common form of birth control in the United States. While there are many different brands and styles of pills, they come in two basic types: combination pills, which contain two kinds of hormones (progestin and estrogen), and progestin only. In combination pills, the user will take pills containing hormones for twenty-one days in a row, followed by seven days of no pills, or seven days in which non-hormone-containing pills can be taken (most packs of pills give you these fake pills so that you stay in your routine of taking a pill every day). During these seven days of fake pill time, menstrual bleeding (your period) occurs. In progestin-only pills, your period is not as predictable; however, some prefer this type of pill because it has fewer side effects.

It's important to take the pill every day at the same time in order for it to be most effective; this is why many women decide to take them either right when they wake up or at night before they go to bed to help remind them (as long as

About Margaret Sanger

Margaret Sanger, a nurse living in America in the early 1900s, was one of the first people to fight for women's rights to birth control. Back in the 1900s, there were strict laws that banned birth control information, and Sanger dedicated her life to fighting this censorship. In 1916, she opened the first birth control clinic and, as a result, was arrested and sent to prison. After her release, she continued the fight to create legal access to birth control. In 1939, Sanger began the Birth Control Federation of America, which later became Planned Parenthood. In the 1950s, her efforts made it possible to find research funding for the first birth control pill.

they have a regular sleep schedule!). Setting a routine is a great way to remember to take the pill consistently. There are also pill-reminder apps available for your phone as well.

Birth Control Pill Summary

How it works: The synthetic hormones in the pills prevent the user from ovulating and the sperm from traveling effectively.

What makes it a good choice: It's private and convenient.

Why it might not be right for you: You may not remember to take the pill at the same time every day. The pill provides no protection against STDs.

How to get it: A doctor gives you a prescription, usually for a year. Then you need to go to the pharmacy every month to get refills. However, some states are now passing laws that allow you to buy birth control pills over the counter directly from the pharmacy.

Cost: Depending on health insurance, the pill costs anywhere from nothing to ninety dollars a month.

Wait time until it works: It takes two to four weeks, depending on the last time you have had your period. Most clinics will suggest using a backup method for a month just to be safe.

How well does it work: It fails less than 1 percent of the time if taken daily at the same time. But no one's perfect; typical failure rate is 9 percent.

In the News

In Oregon and California, birth control pills can be obtained directly from pharmacies over the counter, without a doctor's prescription. In Oregon you have to be at least eighteen years old; California doesn't have an age restriction. Washington and Colorado are considering similar policies to allow over-the-counter access of birth control pills.

What can go wrong: You can forget to take it, making the chances of pregnancy increase significantly.

Question:

I have been on birth control pills for about a year and a half. Does the effectiveness of the pill ever wear down?

—Twenty-two-year-old in Virginia

Answer:

No it does not. Sometimes your cycles can vary after years on the same pill, but you never lose effectiveness as long as you take them on a regular basis.

No worries,

Dr. X, We Are Talking, teen health website

Question:

What are the chances of getting pregnant while you are on your period and on birth control, considering that you don't take your birth control for the days you are menstruating?

—Eighteen-year-old

Answer:

It's important to take the pills every day at the same time, or there is a chance of pregnancy. You should not get pregnant on the days you are not taking the pill because you are having a period (meaning that you ovulated before your period started), and although the sperm can live in your body several days, you will start taking the pills again, and should be protected. If you have missed a period, you can do a home urine pregnancy test, which is the same as those done by physicians' laboratories. Test the urine from the first time you urinate in the morning, when the urine is the most concentrated and would have the most pregnancy hormone to detect (called HCG). You can do the test at least one day after your period has been late.

Great Question,

Dr. X, We Are Talking, teen health website

Other Pill Facts

If you forget to take a pill, it's possible that you could become pregnant. If you forget to take one pill (in other words, miss one day), take it as soon as you remember and take your next pill at the usual time. If you miss two pills in a row, take two pills the day you remember and two pills the next day. After that, go back to your regular schedule. If you forget three in a row, call a health-care professional for instructions and use a backup method until you and your health-care provider decide that your pills are effective again.[1]

Don't want your period on a particular month? All is not lost when you are on the pill. Being on the pill allows you to control when you get your period. If the vacation you have planned falls on the very same week that your period is supposed to come, simply do not take your "fake reminder" pills and immediately start your next pack. That way, you will not get your period at all that month. It's perfectly healthy to do this every once in a while.[2]

If you get sick, there are certain antibiotics that make the pill less effective. If you are given prescription medication because you are sick, tell your doctor you are on the pill so that she makes sure to warn you of any possible drug interactions.

Depo-Provera

Depo-Provera is a shot that needs to be given by a doctor every twelve weeks (three months). The shot contains progestin, which prevents ovulation so there is no egg that can be fertilized; the progestin also slows down the sperm.

Depo-Provera Summary

How it works: The Depo-Provera shot injects progestin, which prevents pregnancy from occurring.

What makes it a good choice: It's private and provides worry-free birth control for months at a time.

Why it might not be right for you: You don't like needles. Your period may change while using the shot. For some women, their periods become non-existent. For others, their periods get heavier or there might be spotting. The shot provides no protection against STDs. You have to go to the doctor every three months to get shots.

How to get it: A doctor gives you the shot every three months.

Cost: It costs up to $120 per shot.

Wait time until it works: After the first shot it takes two to four weeks, depending on the last time you had your period.

How well does it work: Very well—as long as you get your next shot on time!

What can go wrong: You don't get the next shot on time, creating pregnancy risk.

Question:

How long does it take for your first Depo shot to be effective?
—Seventeen-year-old

Answer:

Depo is not instantly effective. You should continue to use a barrier method contraception, like condoms, for the first month after the shot. After that, if you get your shots when you should, then you will continue to be protected against pregnancy.

Remember, Depo-Provera alone will not protect you from sexually transmitted diseases (STD).

Dr. X, We Are Talking, teen health website

The Ring

The ring (a.k.a. NuvaRing) is a small plastic circle that contains progestin and estrogen. It's inserted into the vagina like a tampon (but without the applicator) every three weeks, and then taken out during the fourth week so that a period can happen. However, if you keep the ring in for four weeks, and then place a new one in right away, you won't have a period. Whether you keep the ring in for three or four weeks, just make sure you put in a new ring every four weeks in order to keep the supply of hormones in your body. The hormones in the ring prevent ovulation. Note: If you get a supply of rings, they need to be stored in the refrigerator if you are going to keep them for more than four months. There is some concern about the ring increasing the risk of blood clots, but these cases are rare. Also, you should not use the ring if you smoke. Talk to a health-care provider about these concerns before considering the ring (you need to get a prescription for it anyway).

Ring Summary

How it works: The synthetic hormones prevent a woman from ovulating and the sperm from getting to the egg.

What makes it a good choice: It's private and convenient.

Why it might not be right for you: You might not be able to remember to put a new ring in. It provides no protection against STDs.

How to get it: A doctor gives you a prescription, usually for a year. Then you need to go to the pharmacy to get refills.

Cost: Depending on health insurance, it can cost up to seventy-five dollars a month.

Wait time until it works: Most clinics will suggest using a backup method for a month just to be safe.

How well does it work: It is the same as birth control pills—it fails less than 1 percent of the time if used perfectly (you change it on time, always put in a new one). Typical use has a failure rate of 9 percent.

What can go wrong: You forget to change the ring or put a new one in.

The Patch

The patch is a thin square that looks like a Band-Aid. It is put on the body, where it will release estrogen and progestin in order to prevent ovulation; the hormones will also thicken cervical mucus to slow down sperm. A new patch needs to be put on every week. Unfortunately, they only come in one color (light beige), so depending on your skin tone, you might want to put it somewhere where it looks less obvious.

Patch Summary

How it works: The synthetic hormones prevent a woman from ovulating and the sperm from getting to the egg.

What makes it a good choice: It's as easy as a Band-Aid!

Why it might not be right for you: You might not remember to change the patch weekly. There is only one color option. The patch provides no protection against STDs.

How to get it: A doctor gives you a prescription, usually for a year. Then you need to go to the pharmacy to get refills.

Cost: Depending on health insurance, it can cost up to eighty-five dollars a month.

Wait time until it works: Most clinics will suggest using a backup method for a month just to be safe.

How well does it work: It is the same as birth control pills—it fails less than 1 percent of the time if used perfectly (you change it on time, always put on a new one). Typical use has a failure rate of 9 percent.

What can go wrong: You forget to put a new patch on, increasing the chances of an unplanned pregnancy.

Implant (Nexplanon)

The implant is a tiny rod, about the size of a match stick, which is placed underneath the skin. There, it releases progestin, which prevents the ovaries from releasing eggs; the progestin also thickens cervical mucus, which helps block sperm. Once a health-care provider puts the implant in, it's good for up to three years. One side effect of the implant is a higher chance of irregular bleeding; in some users, periods get a lot lighter or may stop.

Implant Summary

How it works: The synthetic hormones prevent a woman from ovulating and the sperm from getting to the egg.

What makes it a good choice: It lasts for years and is very effective.

Why it might not be right for you: You might not like the idea of having something under your skin. It provides no protection against STDs.

How to get it: A doctor puts it in.

Cost: Depending on health insurance, it can cost up to $800 including the visit.

Wait time until it works: Most clinics will suggest using a backup method for a month just to be safe.

How well does it work: It's one of the most effective options.

What can go wrong: Not much.

So now you have read about all the different contraceptive options available to you. Table 6.1 provides a summary that shows how effective each is when used perfectly and typically.

Emergency Contraception

The condom breaks, the diaphragm slips, two people have vaginal sex without birth control for whatever reason, or there is nonconsensual sex. If pregnancy is

Table 6.1. Proportion of Pregnancies over One Year of Use

Method	Perfect Use	Typical Use
Implant	.05	.05
IUD	.2	.2
Depo-Provera	.2	6
Birth control pill	.3	9
Ring	.3	9
Patch	.3	9
Diaphragm	6	12
Sponge	9	12
Condom	2	18
Natural family planning	5	24
Spermicide	18	28
Chance	85.0	85.0

Source: Guttmacher Institute, "Contraceptive Use in the United States," updated October 2015, https://www.guttmacher.org/sites/default/files/factsheet/fb_contr_use_0.pdf. Accessed May 20, 2016.

a concern, there is a solution called emergency contraception. Emergency contraception (EC) is a pill that provides the body with a one-time intense dose of hormones, upsetting the normal fertility cycle. This sudden hormonal change will decrease the chances of a pregnancy from occurring for up to five days, but the sooner it is taken the more effective it is at preventing a pregnancy.

One kind of EC, Plan B, is available over the counter without a prescription. However, not all pharmacies offer it so it's better to call in advance. You can also buy EC online to have on hand so you are prepared for the unexpected (go to www.not-2-late.com to find EC near you).

Without using emergency contraception, 8 percent of women who have unprotected intercourse during the second or third week of their menstrual cycle will become pregnant. With emergency contraception, only 2 percent will become pregnant. Taking emergency contraception can be rather unpleasant, causing nausea and dizziness. But for most, it's better to feel yucky for a couple of days than to risk being pregnant.

It's important to remember that emergency contraception is exactly what it says it is—it is something to be used in an emergency. If you are having vaginal sex, you need to have a different form of birth control that you use regularly other than this. Taking EC often can be taxing on the body and the soul, so it should not be used as a primary form of contraception. That said, EC can be a very effective way to prevent an unplanned pregnancy, so knowing how to access it is a good thing to think about before you really need to.

RELATIONSHIPS

Relationships are a very important part of human life. Healthy relationships help babies grow faster and stronger, help people have better self-esteem, and make communities safer places to live. One example that illustrates how people need human contact is an experiment that was conducted in the 1940s. Babies in an orphanage were raised in two different ways. The first group of babies were fed and bathed and clothed, but otherwise were raised in isolation in order to prevent them from catching any infectious diseases. Feeding took place in the crib with a propped-up bottle. There was little social give-and-take, little talk, little play.

The second group of babies was raised in a group setting where there was a lot more social stimulation. They were held when fed, attended to when they cried, and played with on occasion. After three or four months, the babies in these two groups began to differ from one another. The babies in the first group became withdrawn and expressionless. They rocked themselves, holding their bodies close to themselves. Some babies even got sick, even though the staff at the orphanage could find nothing wrong with them. From this study, researchers have concluded that people need human contact simply in order to survive. In other words, humans need relationships.[1]

However, many people have taken the need for relationships to the extreme. They believe that they absolutely need to be in a romantic relationship in order to be somebody, feel loved, or simply "fit in" with the rest of the world. In short, there are people out there who believe they are nothing without a significant other. Sure, being in a relationship may make you feel as though you belong, as though you are wanted, loved, and desired, but everybody is a somebody regardless of relationship status. And rarely are we truly alone in this world: we have family, friends, community, and/or other forms of support.

Wanting to be in a relationship simply in order to feel better about yourself and your social status has an effect on your relationship—a bad effect. The desire to be in a relationship just to make you more popular, get into a new set of friends, or feel as though you belong will influence the expectations you have on your relationship. You may believe that simply being in a relationship will make you more popular, help you feel better about yourself, and make you more mature. A relationship cannot do all those things. Such unrealistic expectations are not met

> **Fact**
>
> ● Those teens who are always in a relationship, bouncing from one person to the next, report not being as happy in their relationships as those who enjoy being single from time to time.[a] So, while relationships can be important, there are benefits to being un-partnered every once in a while, too!

and end up placing a strain on the true bond between two people. Whether or not you are in a relationship, you are still going to be you. Liking yourself outside the relationship is essential in order to have great friends and a great significant other at some point in your life.

Reasons to Be in a Relationship with Someone

Out of all the different reasons a person would want to go out with another, there are two basic types. The first type is a personal reason. Personal reasons concern you and your partner only. There is no consideration of anyone else in your decision to date each other. If you are dating someone because you like that person's personality, looks, and other characteristics, the two of you get along well together, and you like and respect each other, then you are dating for personal reasons.

The second type is social. Social reasons consider other people and how they think about you or the person you are with. So, if you are dating someone because that person is popular, so that you will be invited to the "right" parties, or simply because you think only unpopular or unattractive people stay single, then you are dating for social reasons.

The bottom line is that relationships are more successful if they happen for reasons that are personal to the people involved in them and are not determined by social pressures.

How can you tell if you are interested in being in a relationship for personal as opposed to social reasons? Do the following exercise and see!

Your Dream Comes True

OK, I want you to imagine you can go out with anyone you want for a day. I mean *anyone* (Beyoncé? Sure, why not?). Imagine you are with that person, and it's the most perfect day ever. You two are having an amazing time. Get a good picture of that person and your day together. Imagine what you would do together (don't get

Movie Reviews: True Love Edition

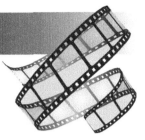

Here are some movies that can help you think about what it means to truly love another person and how being in love can also mean facing challenges as a couple:

- *Save the Last Dance* (2001, 1h 52m): Can a white suburban girl with hopes of being a ballerina really be a good match for a popular black hip-hop dancer?
- *The Notebook* (2004, 2h 4m): A country boy and rich heiress fall in love, but her family totally disapproves and encourages her to become engaged to someone of her status. In the end, love prevails through years of separation, war, and sickness.
- *The Fault in Our Stars* (2014, 2h 13m): Two cancer survivors fall in love as they search for the author of their favorite novel.

---

too excited now . . .). You will always remember that day as the most perfect day with this completely gorgeous, wonderful person. Picture the person that will be with you on your perfect date.

Now there is a catch to this perfect date. (Of course! There is always a catch!) You can't tell anyone about it. And if you do try to tell someone—anyone—about it, no one will believe you. In fact, if you try to tell anyone about it, you will be the laughingstock of your friends and your school. How does the catch to the story make you feel? Does it change the person you want to be with? Why or why not?

Going through this imaginary exercise might help you figure out if you are more interested in dating a particular someone for personal or social reasons. If you were annoyed when you heard the catch to the story, or said to yourself, "Then what is the point of being with that person?" chances are you want to be with that person for social reasons. If you still choose the same person, despite the catch to this game, congratulations! You are probably choosing that person for personal reasons—and that's the start to a healthy relationship.

Crushes

What the heck is a crush anyway? At some point in time, most of us have had one or two. Or thirty-seven. We know it, feel it, when we have one, but crushes are pretty hard to define. To me (a renowned crush expert in my day), having a crush on someone is falling in "love" with a person you don't really know, or being attracted to someone without that person knowing about your feelings. Getting a crush on someone is actually pretty easy— you don't even have to get to know the person you have a crush on. I mean, how many people get crushes on celebrities and never even see them in real life (no way I am the only one out there)? How many times is a particular name scribbled on a piece of paper over and over again during a particularly boring class? Yup—crushes are everywhere and can happen to anyone.

But even though *getting* a crush is easy, oftentimes *having* a crush is tough. Sure, it may be fun at first to see if you can "accidentally" run into your crush at school, or at the mall, or at a party. It might be fun to follow your crush on Facebook or Instagram and comment on a lot of your crush's stuff. A simple smile or "like" from this person can send you into utter bliss for hours. But, after a while, all of this can get pretty tiring and difficult. You want the person to know how you feel, but are paralyzed by the fear of rejection. The pain might start to eat away at your very soul. The obsession you have with this person may even start to interfere with friendships, schoolwork, or other activities. As soon as a crush starts to hurt, it has gone bad.

The reason crushes don't usually last long, and are not satisfying, is that they are not real relationships. Sure, the feelings that come along with a crush can be very real, but the relationship is not. First of all, there is often no relationship at all (take, for example, the celebrity crush—talk about someone not knowing you exist!). Second, the feelings a person has when having a crush on someone are not always based in reality. Emotions are based not on an actual person, but on what that person believes the crush should be like, or wants them to be like. What I mean by this is, if you have a crush on someone, it's almost impossible to see the real person you are attracted to—you put that person on a pedestal. A crush has no faults. A crush can do no wrong. A crush is a perfect specimen of a human being.

But crushes are people. And all people have faults and flaws: these are what can make someone more interesting and complex. It's important to remember that. In fact, when someone has a crush on another, it's sometimes a good idea for that person to get to know the crush as much as possible. Learn about that person's good points, but also the not-so-good points. Know that this person has faults, just like anyone else. Know that your crush is different from you and different from the image you have of that person in your mind. Know that your crush might have different opinions, fashion style, habits and interests than you would wish for. By personalizing crushes, you put them back in their place—on earth, where they belong. You may really like the real person hidden behind your adoration, or you may decide that this person is not someone you are interested in romantically or sexually after all.

Learning about the person behind the crush can be relatively easy if that person goes to your school or lives near you—though sometimes it can feel scary. Try saying "hi" or doing something together, even if it's just science lab or homework. Leave messages on your crush's wall or send a thoughtful text to see how and if that person reacts. Actually get to know the person you have been admiring from afar. If you still like that person—imperfections and reality and all—that's great; hopefully that person will like you back. If you don't like that person, that's OK too. Seeing people as they are is the best way to have a good relationship with someone special—different, imperfect—but still special to you.

Starting a Relationship

Starting a relationship is difficult, to say the least. It requires a lot of guts to take that first step in order to figure out if someone is interested in you the way you are interested in that person. Often, this relationship-starting stuff happens online first, where it feels safer. Especially if you are shy, you might try to get to know someone better by spending time together on social media. You might comment a lot on things this new person in your life has to say, or post funny messages on that person's wall. If that person has any interest in you, you will get a response back. The person might be doing it as a friend, or because there are mutual feelings of attraction and interest.

This online communication can go back and forth for a while, but at some point it's probably a good idea to meet up in person and talk with each other to see if you click. The image that a person presents online can be a little different than when the two of you are chatting face-to-face, and you want to make sure the vibe and feelings are still there when you two are hanging out together. Sometimes attractions that exist online can disappear when you are with someone in person—and it's also true that someone you aren't really drawn to online can be more appealing when you are together. Spending time with a person in a group or one-on-one can probably give you a sense as to whether you want to see if there is couple potential.

Then, at some point, you might want to ask someone out, or see if someone you like has a romantic and/or sexual interest in you. If that's how you're feeling, go for it! Asking someone out isn't easy, and there is a chance it won't work out, but here are a few tips:

- Ask someone when the two of you are alone. You don't need a bunch of friends hanging around listening in on your private conversation.
- Ask someone face-to-face. Texts and messages aren't the right place to see if there is true relationship potential.

- Have an idea as to what you are asking the person before asking! Are you asking someone out on a date? To be a couple? To mess around? Being clear about what you want and asking for it is a good way to start a relationship—or stop it before you both get too confused as to what is going on.

If you ask someone out and that person says no, that's OK. Sure it hurts, but it happens. It happens to everyone. Just say "Oh well," or "Bummer," or whatever and go find a friend or someone who can distract you or remind you of what an amazing person you are. And if someone asks you out and you say no, do it nicely. Say, "No thank you," and maybe provide a small reason—you aren't interested in

---

Youth Speak Out: Asking Someone Out, by Rodney

Have you ever loved someone or "like-liked" someone? You know, when you get that warm feeling whenever you're around them, and you get butterflies whenever you talk to them, maybe sometimes stutter and act odd? Don't worry; we all are like that at some point or another. It's completely natural. But it's also difficult to express your feelings to said person, so they may never know that you're interested in them. That's why you gotta step up and let them know how you feel.

If you get rejected, trust me, it's not the end of the world. You can trust me, a random stranger, because I've been there, quite a few times in fact. It makes you stronger in the end, and makes finding "the one" all the more sweeter. I think. I dunno yet. We'll just say it does for the sake of sounding optimistic. Love is an odd thing, right? You're pretty much pouring your heart out to this one person who you have decided that you care about a ton. Probably why it "hurts" so bad to get rejected, to not have the feeling returned. I personally find it's hard to stay friends with someone after you've poured your heart out to them and they're like "Neat. Go away." (Yes, that actually happened to me once.)

So, if you're in the opposite shoes, take a moment to think about what the person who just professed their love to you has actually done. They've taken the courage and bravery to open up to you and tell you how they feel. For some, explaining how they feel is nearly impossible. Before you turn them down (or accept them) think about how the situation must feel for them. I'm not saying you *have* to like them back, just let them down in a nice way if you have to.[b]

dating, you are already seeing someone, or you just want to stay friends. No need to go on and on about why you are saying no. Someone is giving you a compliment when asking you out or expressing interest in you, even if you aren't interested. It's risky to ask someone out, and it's super difficult to hear a no, even if it's said nicely. A little respect between two people goes a long way.

Healthy Relationships

There is no secret formula that will guarantee a perfect relationship. No strict code to follow, no "to-do" list that will ensure relationship bliss forever. However, when you start to think about the relationship you are in—whether it is or is not working out okay—here are some things to ponder as you try to put your finger on what it is that the two of you need to take the relationship to the next stage:

1. *Your partner.* It sounds pretty basic and obvious, but your partner is an essential part of your relationship. Do the two of you really like each other, or are you just attracted to each other? Is the person you are dating a nice person? Do you like your partner's friends? Interests? If the two of you are not friends, the relationship will not get very far on attraction alone.
2. *Your involvement with each other.* How much time do the two of you spend with each other? How close are the two of you, really? How close do you want to be? A serious relationship takes a lot of time and effort from both people.
3. *The nature of the relationship.* What do the two of you do together? Do you have fun? Truly enjoy each other's company? It takes more than physical attraction to have a true relationship.
4. *Your feelings about and in the relationship.* How does the person you are with make you feel? Happy? Loved? Irritated? Frustrated? Good about yourself? Bad about yourself? In relationships there will always be tough times, but overall the good feelings should outweigh the bad ones.
5. *The future of the relationship.* What do you want to get out of this relationship? A date to the prom? A wedding ring? A best friend? If the two of you have different goals for the relationship, it may be a good idea to clear the air between the two of you and figure out what is best. If each of you wants something that the other does not, it may be best to move on. It's only fair to both of you to respect the needs of the other.

Additionally, there are some important elements that, if not present in a relationship, may cause the bond to weaken instead of strengthen with time. Here are some things that are really important to creating a good relationship with someone. Remember—these things are not enough to keep a couple together, but without them, it's less likely a relationship will last.

Trust

Trust means that you believe in your partner, your relationship, and what is said during the times you communicate with each other. Trust allows each of you to have your own lives, be able to spend time apart, and have close friendships with other people, no matter the gender of that friend. If you trust in each other and the relationship, there will be fewer insecurities, fewer worries, and less jealousy between the two of you.

Respect

Respect means liking your partner for who that person truly is and what that person does. It means being proud of your partner's personality, dreams, and accomplishments. The two of you feel honored and lucky to be seen with one another—not just because of how popular each is, but because each thinks that the other is a great person who has a lot to offer.

Balance and Compromise

When a relationship is healthy, partners spend quality time together and quality time apart. They encourage each other to engage in their own activities and hobbies, even if the other person doesn't find them so interesting. Of course they also do some things together. It is important to share common interests, but it is just as important to have things you do on your own so that each of you is a distinct person without the other.

Sometimes it is hard to balance your together activities with your solo activities. When that happens, the two of you need to talk to each other about what is really important to you. There may be times when you can't do everything you want to do because you need to take your partner's feelings and wishes into consideration. That's where compromise comes into the picture. Sometimes you need to give some of your time, and sometimes you simply need to say to the other that this activity is very important to you and you are willing to sacrifice a different event, but not this one. In a healthy relationship one person is not always the giver and the other the taker. Each needs to do a little of both.

Expressing and Listening

Great relationships involve great communication. If you are not sure how your partner is feeling, ask. If you are feeling particularly happy, sad, or mad about something, talk to your partner about it—even if it has nothing to do with the relationship directly. It's important to share what's going on in your life so that your partner can offer support or check in with you more often if something is challenging you. Your partner can also celebrate your life successes with you. People are not mind readers. Ask each other how you are feeling; find out what matters to your partner. Then, when someone is sharing feelings, concerns, or excitement, it's very important to listen. Put down your cell phone, stop texting, look away from the screen, and look your partner in the eye and really pay attention. By communicating with and listening to each other, a couple is more likely to work out the natural bumps in a relationship and grow together. These actions also show you truly care for the other person. In fact, communicating in a relationship is so important there is a whole chapter on it in this book! See chapter 8 for more on talking and listening to your partner.

Work and Dedication

A healthy relationship takes a lot of time, dedication, and work from both halves of the couple. Without this effort, a couple will begin to take things for granted until the relationship dissolves into nothing. Check in with your partner; make sure you do fun things together. Tell each other how you feel. Appreciate each day you spend together—even the tough ones.

Happiness

Finally, and perhaps most importantly, a relationship should make each person feel happy. Sure, relationships require work and compromise, but in the end being in the relationship should bring a sense of joy and comfort.

Things That Can Make a Good Relationship Not-So-Good

Every relationship has challenges—no way can you be with someone for a long period of time without coming up against some difficulties. Hopefully, couples can talk about what's bothering them and work out tough spots as issues come up.

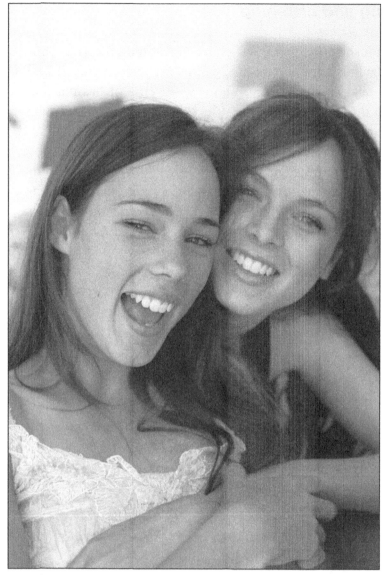

Happiness is a key part of any healthy relationship.

This section mentions some things that can happen in any relationship that can make it take a turn for the worse if they aren't talked about. By acknowledging feelings that you may have with your partner, or with a friend or trusted adult, you may be able to get through some rough times in a relationship.

However, it's important to think about how often these challenges come up in a relationship. If they are happening a lot, and at the expense of all the things that make a relationship great—trust, respect, listening, balance, and happiness—then that could be a sign that the relationship isn't working and that could mean the relationship may need to come to an end. If these challenges are dominating the relationship—or are happening in a way that hurts one person or makes part of the couple feel unsafe—then this is a serious concern. When one or many of these challenges happen consistently, or at a more extreme level, this can be a sign that the relationship is unhealthy, has the potential to become violent, or is maybe already violent. See chapter 9, "Dating and Sexual Violence," for more information about unhealthy relationships.

Jealousy

Jealousy is being afraid that your partner is more interested in someone else than you. Jealousy is being afraid that your partner will leave you when that person shows interest in activities that do not involve you and spending all your time together. Jealousy is pain and suspicion that your partner doesn't care about you.

It's common to feel jealous in a relationship—especially a new one. You have not had time to get to know the person you are dating all that well, and you might feel insecure about where the relationship is going and how much the person you are with really likes you. In this way jealousy is a form of insecurity and is very natural. With time, you should feel less and less jealous in a relationship as the two of you grow closer and learn to trust each other.

If you find that your jealousy or the jealousy of your partner does not decrease with time, then there is a problem. If the two of you have been dating for a while, and there is still suspicion every time someone talks to someone else or spends a lot of time with friends, then that shows there is a lack of trust in the relationship or one person is trying to control the other. A person should be able to interact with people outside of the dating relationship without being constantly checked up on or questioned. Those constant texts asking where someone is or who that person is with are not always signs of caring, but signs of jealousy and insecurity. Being checked up on constantly isn't always a sign of concern; it could be a sign of distrust or a need to control. Without trust, it's very hard to have a successful relationship.

Betrayal

Betrayal means lying and/or cheating on your partner, and most people believe that cheating is not acceptable in a relationship. Not only does cheating hurt the relationship and the feelings of another, but it can also put everyone at increased risk for STDs if unprotected sex is involved.

Many times the person who cheats feels bad about doing it, but that still does not mean it's OK. Cheating can be a sign that the feelings between two people aren't equal—that one person may be taking the relationship more seriously than the other. If you believe that you might cheat on your partner, talk to your partner about being less serious or break off the relationship completely. It's not fair to the other person to do otherwise. If you think you are going to cheat, that is a sign that the relationship may be too serious for you or that the two of you are growing apart. Relationships change over time, and most relationships do not last a lifetime. It's good for both of you to be honest up front about your feelings and maybe step back from the commitment. If you think you are being cheated on, talk to your partner about it. It will be a hard conversation to have, but in the long run, being honest with each other about the commitments you are and are not ready to keep will make your relationships more successful. If you tell someone you are only going to be with him or her, it's important to stay true to your word.

Conflict

In general, there is nothing wrong with conflict in a relationship. In fact, a little bit of conflict in a relationship is a good thing. Getting into an argument or debate with your partner shows that the two of you are being honest with each other and true to yourselves by sharing what you believe, even if those opinions do not match the beliefs of the other. It shows that the two of you, although wonderful together, also have your own thoughts and feelings—you are your own person without the other. When you feel close to someone, it's only natural that you are going to disagree from time to time, and that you are each going to do things that will upset the other in some way. And because you care about each other, and care what the other thinks about you, it makes sense that when a disagreement happens, one or both of you might feel sad and upset. That's OK, too, providing that the two of you work things out together.

   And that's the important part and what makes conflict healthy or not healthy. A great relationship is not about whether a couple has conflict from time to time, but about how the couple deals with conflict when it comes up. The best way to deal with a conflict is to talk about it when both of you are not really upset. Of course, it's normal to feel sad, angry, or irritated with your partner when the two of you disagree. However, this is not the best time to talk about the problem. If the tension is too high, take a step back from the problem, or even from each other, and leave the issue alone for a while. Only when the two of you are both calm and ready to talk will you be able to address the problem rationally and productively. And when you do talk about it again, try to stay calm, really listen to your partner's side of the story, and work on an agreement that both of you think is OK. Just as importantly, make sure your partner is really listening to you and what you have to say. Together, you can hopefully come to an understanding the two of you are OK with. A little give-and-take can go a very long way.

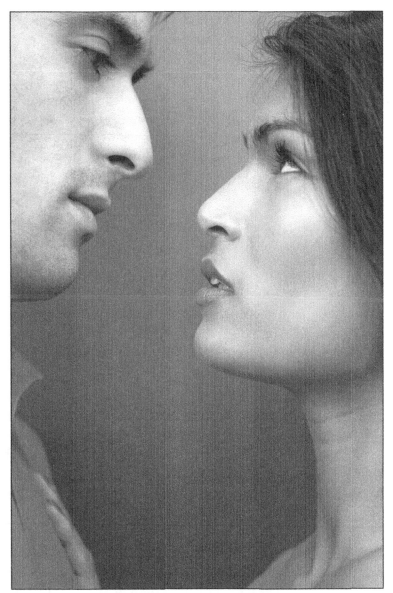

Conflict is a natural part of any relationship, so it's important to disagree in ways that do not involve violence or manipulation.

There are many ways to end an argument that never work:

- *Violence.* Never, never, never hurt someone when you are disagreeing over something (or any other time). You should not hurt someone physically *or* emotionally. Name-calling or delivering a "low blow" to make your partner upset will never resolve an argument, even if you think it will make you feel better in the short term. If you find yourself being hurt during an argument, leave immediately and go to a friend or relative you can trust. For more on this, see the next chapter.

- *Ignoring the problem.* Sure, if one or both of you is really upset, you should forget about the argument—temporarily. But if you do not talk about what happened, the problem will keep coming up again and again until something is really done.
- *Doing all the giving or all the taking.* Without truly listening to the other's side of the argument and working out a compromise, someone's opinions or feelings get shut out. In a good relationship, two people need to work together to make things happen. If someone is always giving in to the other, that person is sacrificing too much just to have a partner.

When a Relationship Ends

It doesn't matter if you do the breaking up, you are broken up with, or the decision is mutual: ending a relationship is difficult and can, frankly, stink. Of course, how you feel might depend on which end of the stick you are on, but then again, it might not matter at all. You will feel some or all of the following: sad, despairing, angry, relieved, insecure, happy, vengeful, strong, weak, alone. It's OK to feel all of these feelings at different times, and even all at once. The key to getting through a breakup is this: no matter how bad it hurts, sucks, overwhelms, or takes over your every thought, it will get better. You will hear many people say that, and you might not believe them and might even get mad at people who say that. But it's true. After a breakup, people get better; they heal and move on when they are ready. Note, I said when they are ready. It may take some time, and it will take some help from friends, relatives, good music, and maybe a counselor, but people survive breakups every day, and so will you.

Although it might be tempting to break it off through text or on social media, it's best to end most relationships in person (providing you believe it's safe to do so). You owe a person you once dated the respect to end the relationship face-to-face. To help you through that nasty breakup time, here is a list of dos and don'ts to consider:

Do write a hate letter or love letter, letting your recent ex know exactly how you feel.

Don't send it or post it online. Instead, print it out and burn it or tear it up as a symbolic end to the relationship. Have a friend witness the burning and make it a celebration of sorts.

Do express the emotions you feel.

Don't lash out at your ex, your friends, your pet, or yourself. Instead, beat a pillow, take a walk, shoot hoops, talk to someone, or let yourself cry.

Do grieve.

Losing Someone You Love

Not all separations happen on purpose. Sometimes tragedy causes a relationship to end when no one is ready. When this happens, I hope you are able to find support in your community and take the time to both grieve and celebrate a relationship that ended too soon. Here is an example of advice I gave to someone who lost a loved one unexpectedly to tragedy.

Dr. Kris,

   My name is Jonatha, and I am a freshman in community college majoring in something, it was nursing, but now, who knows? Anyway, I guess that I am supposed to write to you about my love problems. Well, that's the thing . . . I don't have any. I haven't been in a serious relationship in two years. My ex boyfriend and I were serious for five years. He passed away in a car accident two years ago. It was rough for the longest time. I was supposed to sit next to him at graduation, but he wasn't there. We were supposed to be king and queen of the prom, he wasn't there. I need to get back into the dating game. I am hoping that you could help me.

Hi Jonatha:

   I am so sorry to hear about what has happened to you. I have lost close friends to tragedy, but never a partner, so I can only imagine what it's like. The first few things you need to do involve you and only you. You have to be honest with yourself about whether you are ready to date again. On one level, two years is a long time. On another, it is less than half the time you two were together. If you really want to start dating other people, that is fine. But I hope you are not feeling as though you want to date again simply because you feel you should. Only you can decide when you are ready to feel close to another person.

   Another thing to do is talk to a counselor (does your school have any for free or lower rates?) about your desires to date again, and also about your goals in school, and other parts of your life. A counselor can help you process your grief and support you in working through this unexpected, painful event. Friends and family can be great sources of support too, but a professional can really help you sort through all that has happened. Even though two years have gone by, now is still a good time to work on things. There is no set time for when you need to move on, but if you want to, that is great. Just remember that you have every right to be sad and grieve, and that it is never too long ago to miss someone.

Dr. Kris[c]

Don't grieve 24/7. Give yourself a set block of time every day (thirty minutes at the most!) to obsess and think and wonder about what went wrong. But when that time is over, so is thinking about that relationship until the next day.

Do feel hurt, if that is how you feel.

Don't hurt yourself. If you start to hurt yourself or even feel like you want to hurt yourself, talk to a trusted adult or call a suicide hotline right away. Cutting and other forms of self-harm don't lead to healing in the long run. There are people out there who want to help you and want you around the way you are.

Do think evil thoughts from time to time.

Don't act on them or allow them to dominate your mind. Think about how bad it would be tomorrow if you did.

Do talk to your friends about how you feel.

Don't make your breakup the only thing you talk about. Remember the rest of the cool things that you are all about? Talk about those things, too! You were and are always more than half of a couple.

Do be nice to each other.

Don't try to stay friends right away. Allow for some time apart, to get used to the idea that you are no longer a couple. Being friends right away can be confusing and can be extra painful, too, as feelings get confused. Chill out for a while—unfriend each other on social networks (it's too tempting to constantly check up on your ex's life without you). In time, the two of you might be able to spend time together again, and it will not be totally strange. But if you can't, that's OK, too.

Do take the time and think about what you learned from the relationship. Think about what was good about it and how it helped change you and make you more mature.

Don't beat yourself up about what you shoulda or coulda done. Or think about all the things your ex coulda or shoulda done to make it work.

Don't completely blame yourself or your ex for what happened. The relationship did not work out, and that's OK. Take the time to grieve, learn from it, remember it, and move on.

TALKING AND LISTENING TO YOUR PARTNER

The most important element of a great relationship and a healthy sex life is both simple and challenging at the same time. The secret ingredient is good communication. Talking about sex, your feelings, and your relationships is not easy. It makes you vulnerable and open to a lot of pain, and it can be very embarrassing. But it can also lead to a very rewarding experience. Learning to express yourself to those you care about leads to self-confidence, the ability to be close to others, and better relationships all around.

Consent

Before you do anything sexually with another person, it's very important to make sure that the person you are with wants to share the experience. It's your responsibility to get consent from your partner before starting anything or moving onto a different sexual activity. For example, if you've been making out with someone for a while and want to move on to removing some clothing—yours or your partner's—you need to ask that person first if it's OK to do so. This type of asking is called getting consent, and it's one of the most important things to do when you are with someone.

Consent is hearing a "yes" to sexual activity. It's not the same as hearing "maybe" or "I'm not sure. I guess." It's also not the same thing as not hearing the word *no*. If you don't hear someone say "Yes!" then there is no consent. If someone is under the influence of alcohol or drugs or is passed out, that person cannot give consent. You absolutely should not engage in any sexual activities with someone who cannot actively consent to something. If you start being sexual with someone who is under the influence, and then realize that person isn't really with it, just stop, make sure that person is safe, and say you will text tomorrow. Even if

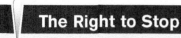

The Right to Stop

• Remember: Everyone has the right to end any sexual activity at any time. As soon as someone wants to stop, the sexual activity must stop.

that person seems to be into what you're doing, there is no consent because there is a lack of complete awareness of what's going on. If you both feel the same way about each other when the two of you are sober, you can pick up where you left off. If feelings change, then you know you did the right thing by stopping.

Asking for consent and hearing a person give consent can be fun. It can be sexy. Knowing—really knowing—another person wants to be doing the same thing you want to do sexually is exciting. It can feel fun, wonderful, loving, amazing. Knowing the person doesn't want to be doing the same thing allows the two of you to stop and find something the two of you want to do together, even if that means stopping the sexual stuff completely. And stopping at the right time can leave you feeling proud, responsible, and caring. If you stop something after not hearing a clear yes, it shows that you are a respectful, mature, and understanding partner. Doing something sexual without knowing for sure that the person you are with is on board with you can lead to hurt feelings, regret, or even sexual assault. Hearing a no and doing something anyway is sexual coercion: it's immoral and illegal.

How do you get consent? Just ask! Here are some examples:

- I would love to kiss you right now. Is that OK?
- I'd feel really sexy if I got undressed. Are you cool with that?
- How are you feeling?
- Is this OK with you?
- What would you like to do right now?
- What would make you feel good?

In order to make sure you have consent at all times, you should check in with the person you are with for every new sexual activity. Anytime you hear someone feeling unsure, or saying no, stop immediately. Go back to what you were doing, or ask if you should stop. Or ask what your partner would like instead. You can ask using a kind, caring tone, or perhaps a sexy tone—or a gentle whisper. But ask. Always ask. Then respect your partner's desires and boundaries. That is the key to consent. Especially in new relationships, it's a good idea to make sure the consent you get is verbal: in other words, make sure you hear your partner say yes each time you start a new sexual activity.

California Says Yes!

In 2015, California governor Jerry Brown signed a law that requires sex education in California to talk about consent through a "yes means yes" standard. Students will be taught that sexual activity is considered consensual only when both partners clearly indicate their desire to participate using "affirmative, conscious and voluntary agreement" for each new sexual activity.[a]

How do you give consent? Easy—just say "Yes!" Or you can say "Heck yeah!" or "I've been thinking about doing that with you for days!" The more enthusiastic and clear, the better. A clear yes shows your partner that you are happy to be with her or him, and that can make both of you feel good. Say yes anytime you really want to do something—not just because your partner wants to do it, or you are feeling pressured for any reason into doing something. Own your yes!

Still unsure about what consent is and isn't? That's OK. This is a difficult topic to grasp. Some people have equated asking for consent with offering a guest a cup of tea.[1]

If you offer someone a cup of tea and that person says, "Yes, please," you make one and see if cream or sugar is desired. Your guest responds, and you make the tea according to those wishes. However, it is possible that during the time it takes for the water to heat up and the tea to steep, your guest will decide tea isn't desired anymore—and that's OK. You simply don't serve tea, even if it was already prepared. Similarly, if your guest falls asleep while you are making tea, you don't serve it, you don't wake your guest up to drink it, and you certainly don't pour it down your sleeping guest's throat! You just put the tea aside and make sure your guest is comfortable and leave it at that. Bottom line: You don't pressure someone into drinking tea; you ask your guest if tea is wanted, and then how you should make the tea. You are cool with your guest deciding tea isn't wanted after all, even if you started making it. Same thing goes for sex—don't do anything your partner doesn't want, and allow your partner to say no anytime.

Talking about Your Relationship with Your Partner

First of all, you can't tell someone how you feel, or what you want in a relationship, if you don't know yourself. It's important to take time out for yourself to think about you and what you want. What are your values? What is important to you in a relationship? What are your sexual boundaries? Your sexual desires? Knowing these things about yourself makes it possible to express them to others. It will still be difficult, but at least you know what the honest answer will be to these important questions.

Once you have a good understanding about what you do and do not want when it comes to having a relationship with someone, it's a good idea to tell that person. Communicating your thoughts and feelings requires two important parts: talking and listening. Therefore, when someone feels ready to talk, that person also should be ready to listen. Both need to happen for communicating to be effective and for two people to understand each other.

Even though it might be hard, it's a good idea to be open and honest about what you are thinking and how you are feeling about someone. If you are in a relationship, it's a good idea to tell that person what you are and are not comfortable with sexually and romantically—and it's important to listen carefully and respectfully when your partner is telling you these things. Without communicating these basic but very important points, a relationship cannot last.

Timing

There are good times and bad times to bring up a conversation about sex and relationships. The best times to talk about serious things like being together or what does and does not feel good in the relationship either emotionally or sexually

What If You Aren't in a Relationship?

There are mixed reviews about whether you should tell someone how you feel when you are not in a relationship with that person. If the person is showing signs of interest in you, then it might be a good idea to break the ice and confess some feelings. But if the person tends to shy away from you, then even if that person does return your feelings, it might not be the right time. One word of advice—even if you believe you are madly in love with someone you do not have a relationship with, it's best not to spill all your feelings at once. Open up slowly, and give both of you a chance to get to know each other.

are times when both of you feel calm, happy, relaxed, and safe. In other words, good times are:

- When the two of you are alone
- When the sun is shining and you can take a walk together
- When you are feeling good and secure about yourself

The not-so-good times to talk are when either of you is not focused or there are a lot of distractions. When neither one of you is able to think clearly, it's easy to not listen carefully or concentrate the way the topic of conversation deserves. Examples of bad times to communicate about your relationships are:

- While texting during class
- If either (or both) of you is drunk or high
- When either (or both) of you is very angry or sad
- When one of you has to leave for an important obligation in less than half an hour
- Late at night when you might be too tired to think clearly

Picking a good time to talk is just as important as knowing what to say. A person cannot respond to your thoughts and feelings if too distracted to hear them or you are too upset to express them coherently!

Listening to a Whole Person

Clear communication is a critical component of a healthy romantic and sexual life. It's important, when you are listening to someone, to listen completely—this means listening to the words you hear and also paying attention to a person's body language. People communicate with and without words. Table 8.1 has some examples.

Sometimes, these different ways of communicating contradict each other. For example, there may be a person who flirts with you all the time, puts an arm around you and all that, but then says no when you ask that person out. Even though you thought the person was sending all the "right" signals, listening to

---

Fact

● About half of young people discuss contraception or sexually transmitted diseases with their partners before having sex for the first time. African American youth were more likely to talk about safer sex than other young people.[b]

Table 8.1. Ways to Communicate

With Words	Without Words
Texting	Body language
Notes	Eye contact
Arguing	Touch
Tone of voice	Personal space/distance

and honoring the words is important. Or someone might say, "I care about you," but then never makes eye contact with you or always has an excuse when you try to get together. This sort of mixed communication can be frustrating when you are trying to figure out how someone feels about you. If this happens and you are confused, try to talk about certain issues directly with that person. Give specific examples so that person understands your point of view. At the same time, you should also think about the ways you are communicating with someone; are they consistent? If your messages are not consistent, try to do your best to change your ways of communicating so that they are consistent with your feelings. Honoring your feelings shows that you have respect for yourself and other people.

For the most part, the best ways to communicate something you feel very strongly about are with words and in person, so that tone can be heard and body language can be seen. No one is a mind reader—if we do not tell anyone what is going on inside of our head, chances are no one will understand how we are feeling. Similarly, if we try to have a serious conversation in messenger or by texting, it's hard to tell what some words mean—whether a person is feeling hurt, mad, confused, or happy. While emojis can help, they aren't perfect. The less personal the mode of communication, the higher the chance of miscommunication and the more likely someone can get confused or hurt over the situation. It's important to remember that people should make decisions about their relationships as a part of a couple, and ideally in a face-to-face setting so there is a better chance that each person understands the other.

Communicating What You Want

In the same way that it's important to listen to someone so that you understand what that person wants, it's also important to communicate what you want. This

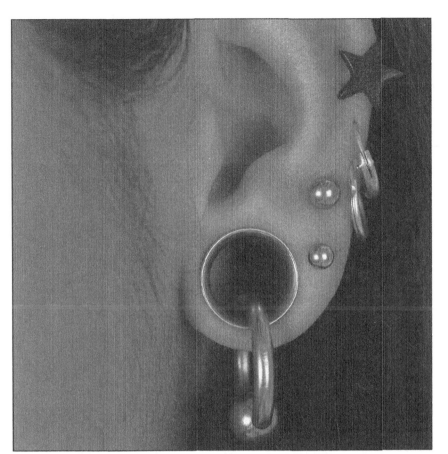

Really listen when your partner expresses feelings or just wants to chat.

sounds pretty obvious, but it can be difficult. Telling someone what you want or need in a relationship can leave you feeling pretty vulnerable. This is because you are being honest with someone about what truly matters to you, and it's scary to risk being rejected or not heard on a very deep level. As with any serious communication, when you want to tell someone something important, do it when the two of you have a lot of time together. Find a quiet spot and face each other to show how serious you need to be about something. Or you can maybe hold hands and look away if it's too difficult to talk face-to-face. You can start the conversation by letting your partner know how hard it is to say what you need to say. Start by saying, "I'm nervous to talk about this, but I feel it's important," or take a deep breath to calm your nerves. If you want to talk about something negative, you can start with a positive first. For example, say, "I really like you, but I miss my friends. I would like to spend more time with them." Then, listen to what your partner has to say. Hopefully, the two of you will be able to talk about things and come to a conclusion that works for the two of you. It may take more than one conversation, but it will be worth it in the end to know you have expressed yourself and have stayed true to what matters to you.

When you are being intimate with someone, it's also great to communicate what you want. You can tell someone what you like by reacting positively to something by saying, "Oh, I really like that," "That feels really good," or "Mmmm. More of that please." Or, you can also state what you like up front: "I love it when you . . . " or "I think it feels really good when you . . ." Simply put, if you like something, tell your partner; if you don't like something, tell your partner! Think about it—you would want to know if what you were doing was making your partner feel good or not. Your partner wants to make you feel good as well.

The Need to Communicate

Check out this story written by someone who can't tell what is going on in her romantic life. What do you think is going on?

At my school dance I went with my best friend Ron. So my friend Maria went with her boyfriend Jose. And well I dared them to kiss cuz they never do. So they did it and then Maria said I had to kiss Ron. And me and him looked at each other. He said, "Maria that's different cuz you two are going out. We are best friends." Well I did it cuz the only person Ron will listen to is me.

So then after that Maria and me ran away to talk. But when we would turn around there would be Jose or Ron. So I said, "You guys stop being hound dogs!" and they both stopped.

Well anyway I have asked Ron out lots of times and he has said no. Then the DJ started to play slow songs so Maria made me and Ron dance. Well we did and after that dance me and Ron were holding hands. Before I left the dance me and Ron hugged. Does he really like me? I mean he has said no to me so many times. We talk on the phone every night. He knows my school schedule by heart. Basically he knows it better than I do. And I've never told him it. When me and Maria would switch coats at school he begged me not to switch coats. Cuz he didn't like going up to Maria in the halls.

Ron's sister hates me cuz she says I call too much and I said uh no its the other way around. He calls me I just return them. I need to know does he like me or what? Or is he just obsessed with me? My friend writes on my hand, "I <3 Ron" everyday on my hand and he knows it. He knows how much I care and love him. But now I think he feels the same about me too.[c]

What do you think?

1. Did these two people get consent from each other to kiss? To dance?
2. To me, these two have a lot to talk about. What do you think they need to sort out before they think about having a relationship?

Setting and Respecting Boundaries

You always have the right to say no to any sexual activity you do not want to do. You have the right to say no anytime you don't want to do something. Sometimes, people are not respectful of your boundaries and these are times when communication needs to become a one-way conversation. Even after doing this, if something happens that you did not want to happen, it is not your fault. If you believe your wishes are not being heard or respected, or if you are feeling pressured to have sex or do something you do not want to do, here are ways to try to get yourself out of a situation you don't want to be in.

Think It Over

Someone may ask you to hang out or express interest in doing something sexually with you, and you aren't sure how you feel about it. That's OK—we don't always know the answer to something right away. Thinking it over means telling someone you need to think about something first before you actually do it. This strategy is all about taking time for yourself so you can think about something first. As was discussed earlier, it's important to think about what your sexual desires and boundaries are. It's best to do this sort of thinking in a quiet setting. Think-it-over phrases you can use include the following:

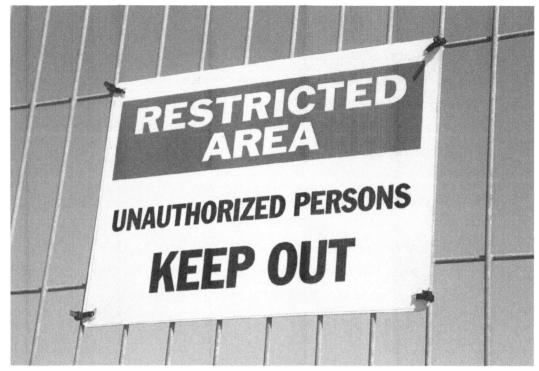

Always respect a person's sexual boundaries.

- "I'll call you back."
- "I'll let you know by [specify day] if that's cool with me."
- "I'm not sure I want to do that. Let me think about it."

Be Firm

Being firm means holding your ground when someone has heard your decision, but for some reason has chosen not to respect your words. You did not give consent and a person still continues to pressure you. A person like this is not to be trusted and, unfortunately, has put you in a position where you have to restate your feelings directly, clearly, and without room for debate. When this happens, it is time to restate your opinion loud and clear and then leave the situation if it is safe to do so.

How to be firm:

- To gain attention, use the name of the person who doesn't seem to be listening.
- Hold up your hand in a firm way and restate your message.
- Repeat what you said in a strong, loud voice, starting with "I said . . ."

How to Respond to a No

It's going to happen in your life—probably several times. Someone is not going to want to do something sexually with you that you want to do. Sure, it's a bummer, but it's also totally normal; people have different interests and different boundaries. And no one owes you anything when it comes to sex. If someone you are with says no to your sexual advances or requests, the right thing to do is simply say, "OK" or "All right. That's fine." Do not ask again, do not ask why, and do not whine, pout, or create any drama (whining and pouting are never sexy). After you say OK, you can ask what that person would like to do instead or if he or she is OK with continuing what you were doing before. If the person isn't sure, just stop what the two of you are doing and give the individual space and time to think. Tell the person you are with that you care and are fine with whatever happens next—you don't want to make anyone feel bad. You want your partner to feel comfortable and safe, and you want to know you are doing the right thing.

Get Away

Sometimes it is best to leave a situation when you feel that talking isn't getting anywhere and you believe it's safe to leave. Sometimes you might want to talk about the situation first by either thinking it over or staying strong. But sometimes your partner will not listen, and other times you might not think that it's worth it. This is when it may be best to just walk away from the situation.

How to get away:

- Get up and leave. If possible, know where you are going.
- Pretend you are about to get sick and bolt.
- Yell "HELP!" (some people say to yell "Fire!" to get attention).
- Call a friend's name who might hear you.

If you are unable to get away from a situation, it is not your fault. See the chapter on sexual violence to learn more.

DATING AND SEXUAL VIOLENCE

No one, absolutely no one, deserves to experience dating or sexual violence. A person who is in a violent relationship did not do anything wrong, nor did that person do anything to cause the violence. A person should not have "known better." It is never the victim's fault if that person ends up in a violent relationship. If you find yourself in a violent relationship, please do not blame yourself for what has happened. This chapter will help you identify warning signs and outline the facts and your rights. Dating violence happens among young people and there are many ways to support yourself or a friend if you find that violent relationships are a part of your life.

What Is Dating Violence?

When we think about an abusive relationship, we usually think of someone being physically violent toward another person. However, there are many forms of dating violence. For example, it can happen when one person tries to control the thoughts, beliefs, or behavior of the partner. One person can control the other person through emotional, sexual, or physical mistreatment. An additional form of emotional abuse for people who are gay, lesbian, bisexual, or trans is being outed by a partner (or a partner may threaten to out them) at school or to family or friends if their sexual/gender orientation is a secret.

Even though dating violence should never happen, it is very common among young people. One and a half million high school students experience physical abuse by their dating partner each year. One in three young people in the United States experiences physical, sexual, emotional, or verbal abuse from a dating partner. In fact, dating violence is the most common form of violence among youth.[1] This means that if you experience dating violence, you are not alone. Sexual violence can happen to anyone, and it is never that person's fault. Please see the resources at the end of this chapter to seek support if you need it for you or a friend.

When we think of abuse, most of us think about someone hitting another. Although this behavior is certainly abusive, there are other ways that a partner can abuse another. Sometimes, these behaviors are on a continuum or path. In other words, one type of violence may lead to another type; for example, a relationship may be emotionally abusive at first, and then also become sexually or physically abusive. Other times someone may be emotionally or physically violent toward a partner, but not both. Usually, the violence is repetitive in an abusive relationship and gets worse over time. It's important to understand all different types of dating violence so that you can recognize them in your own relationships or your friends' relationships.

Emotional Violence

Emotional violence or abuse is when someone tries to control another person through words and actions. This control can be really subtle and can be combined with statements like, "I'm just saying this because I love you" or "I'm only doing this because I care about you and want to protect you." This can make the control hard to identify, because it comes with mixed messages. However, one way to tell the difference between kindness and emotional abuse is that a person who is being emotionally abusive often makes the partner feel ashamed, insecure, meaningless, ugly, or afraid. There are many ways a person can be emotionally abusive. Here are only a few:

- Calling a partner names like *stupid*, *slut*, *fat*, or *useless*, in order to make the partner feel bad
- Constantly checking up on a partner's whereabouts—even after that person has already communicated plans
- Posting mean messages about a partner even if only in jest
- Checking a partner's cell phone to see whom the person has been communicating with
- Continually threatening to leave
- Cheating on a partner and then blaming those actions on something the partner did, instead of admitting any wrongdoing
- Threatening suicide if the partner leaves
- Laughing at or humiliating a partner in front of others
- Accusing a partner of being interested in other people, and feeling very jealous every time a partner talks to someone else

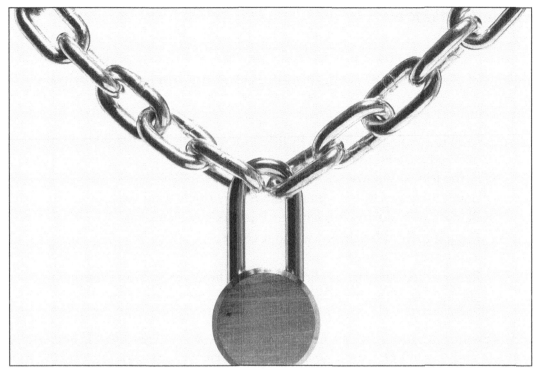

Emotional abuse includes being isolated from others and being controlled.

- Wanting to spend every waking minute with a partner to the point of isolating that person from family and friends

Physical Violence

Physical violence or abuse is when a person causes bodily harm to another. It can also mean doing something physical that indirectly hurts a partner. The ways people are physically abusive include:

- Hitting
- Punching
- Throwing someone against a wall
- Throwing things near a person, so that they just miss
- Pulling hair
- Throwing someone out of a car
- Stealing or breaking someone's favorite possessions
- Getting someone hooked on drugs or alcohol
- Squeezing or grabbing someone so tightly that it hurts

Sexual Violence

Sexual violence or abuse is when someone does something sexually to another that isn't wanted, or without consent. The ways people are sexually abused include:

- Having their butt, breasts, or other personal part of the body grabbed or touched without consent
- Being forced to have sex (oral, anal, or vaginal)
- Being forced to watch sexual videos they don't want to see
- Being filmed during sex without knowledge or consent
- Having their sexts shared without consent
- Being sent unwanted sexts
- Being called sexually explicit names without permission ("cat calling")
- Having sex without protection even after they insisted on it

Sexual violence affects all of us in different ways. One out of four young women and one out of twenty young men experiences sexual assault by the time they are seventeen years old.[2] If sexual abuse happens to you, you are not alone. Those people in your life may or may not come forward or let you know what has happened to them, but the bottom line is this: we all know someone, if not many people, who have experienced sexual violence. Please use the resources at the end of this chapter to support yourself or someone else who has experienced sexual violence and wants help.

What Is Rape?

Rape is a type of sexual violence where sexual intercourse happens without consent. Rape can happen when sex is coerced, forced, manipulated (that means, someone was tricked into having it), or happens without both people agreeing explicitly to it. Any form of unwanted sex is rape. Remember: Any time something sexual happens, both people need to consent to the activity. Consent is when both people say yes. Silence—not hearing the word *no*—is not consent. Only a no-doubt-about-it yes is consent. A person has a right to say no at any time, even if that person says yes at first. When people say yes, then change their minds to no, consent has been taken away. No does not mean yes, or keep on trying until the person says yes. No means no, and that is the end of it.

Anyone can say no to sex at any time. The following reasons do not justify unwanted sex:

Oscar-Worthy Moment

Vice President Joe Biden spoke out against sexual violence when he introduced Lady Gaga's performance of "Till It Happens to You," a song from the documentary *The Hunting Ground*, a movie about sexual assault on college campuses. During his speech, Biden said, "Let's change the culture. We must and we can change the culture so that no abused woman or man . . . feels like they have to ask themselves, 'what did I do wrong?' They did nothing wrong." To learn more and take a pledge to help stop sexual violence by intervening if you witness a nonconsensual sexual situation, go to ItsonUs.org.

- If a person dresses sexy.
- If a person claims to be so turned on as to not be able to stop or help him- or herself.
- If a person has said yes to sex before—even if that person had sex before with that same person (even minutes before). A person can choose not to have sex with any person at any time, for whatever reason.
- If a person says yes only after being pressured into saying so. The consent needs to be genuine to count and can't come from a place of force or trickery.

Another important thing to remember about consent is that a person has to be aware of what is going on in order to consent to sex. This means that people cannot give consent if they are:

- Drunk
- Asleep
- Mentally or emotionally challenged in a way that limits ability to consent
- Passed out
- On drugs

If someone has sex with a person under any of the conditions listed here, that person has committed rape. For a refresher on consent, go back to chapter 8.

Rape and Sex

• Although rape includes actions that are a lot like sex, rape is not sex. Rape is an act of violence. Rape is an unhealthy expression of power and dominance. Rape is illegal.

There are different types of rape. When people are asked to make up a story about a rape, most will talk about a strange, evil person sneaking up on someone from behind a tree or the shadows of an alley. This type of rape is called stranger rape, and it's an uncommon form of sexual assault. Acquaintance rape happens between two people who know each other. Most reported rapes—70 percent—happen between two people who have met before.[3] Surveys about sexual assault that include both reported and unreported rapes puts that percentage even higher—more than 80 percent.[4] If intercourse without consent happens between two people who are dating, it's sometimes called date rape.

Another type of rape is statutory rape. This type of rape happens if a legal adult has sex with someone under the age of consent. The age of consent is different in every state in the United States, but is always between sixteen and eighteen. It is also different in different countries so it's important to know the age of consent where you live. Even if the sex is consensual (that is, both people agree to have sex with each other), it can still be considered statutory rape if one of the people is underage. This is because the laws are written assuming that people under the age of consent are not able to realize the implications and importance that sex can have on a person's physical and emotional well-being. Therefore, the law was written to protect youth from being taken advantage of by older people.

Rape Drugs

While alcohol is the most commonly used rape drug (see chapter 12 for more information on sex and alcohol), there are other drugs that are also used to lower people's inhibitions, making them more vulnerable to sexual assault and rape. Although it is never a person's fault if that individual is drugged, it is a good idea to know about these substances and their effects in order to know the signs so you can act if you believe you or a friend were given something.

Rohypnol (roofies, rophies, forget pill) and GHB (liquid X, liquid E, liquid ecstasy) are illegal substances that can be used to facilitate a rape. They are also sometimes taken recreationally. It is extremely dangerous to use either of these drugs with alcohol. Mixing alcohol and either of these drugs can result in low blood pressure, difficulty breathing, coma, or even death.

Both Rohypnol and GHB are colorless and odorless. This means that both of these drugs can be dissolved into a drink (alcoholic or not), and it would be difficult to notice. When people consume a "dosed" drink, they will become drowsy and may even lose consciousness. This allows the rapist to take advantage of someone without the fear of that person fighting back. In addition, as these drugs wear off, the person affected often cannot remember what happened, allowing the rapist to have a better chance of getting away with the crime.

One of the signs that you have been drugged is feeling a lot more drunk or intoxicated than you believe you should given the amount of alcohol you have consumed. If you feel this way, find a trusted friend immediately and have that person watch you. Tell that person you may have been drugged, because you are feeling extremely "fuzzy" and confused, and are having a hard time remembering things; if you pass out, that person should take you to a hospital immediately, as the combination of these drugs and alcohol can be fatal. GHB is particularly dangerous because there is a very narrow margin between a dose that will produce intoxication effects and the amount that will lead to serious and harmful effects. Rohypnol can induce a coma and also cause death, so its effects also should not be taken lightly. Don't worry about the consequences of underage drinking—safety is the priority here. It is never your fault if you consume a drink that has been tampered with. In fact, some states have passed laws so that young people will not be charged for their alcohol or drug use if they are reporting sexual violence.

The Warning Signs

Although there are many types of dating violence, there are patterns to look for if you think your partner may be abusive or may have the potential to be abusive. Ask yourself—does your partner:

- Act jealous and possessive toward you? If someone will not let you see or talk to friends and family, if someone constantly follows you or asks you where you have been, that is abusive.
- Text you at all hours of the day or night insisting to know where you are and who you are with?
- Embarrass you by insulting you or calling you names? Your partner could do this in public or in private. Sometimes, when you ask your partner to stop, she or he might accuse you of having no sense of humor, taking things too seriously, or being too sensitive. The truth is, if you do not like

what is happening, your partner should respect your wishes and stop do-ing it.

- Try to control you by giving orders and making all of the decisions? If you offer an opinion, does your partner ignore it or say it's a dumb idea?
- Pressure you to do sexual things that you do not want to do?
- Want to wrestle or pretend fight in a way that hurts you or makes you feel uncomfortable? If you protest, does your partner say you are stupid and complain that you take things too seriously?
- Hit, grab, or push you at any time? It does not matter if the two of you are in an argument or not—physical violence is always wrong.
- Make you feel afraid that you will be hit, or given the silent treatment, or made to feel bad in some other way—making you feel that it's your fault if your partner is mad?

These are also warning signs you can think about if you are worried you might be abusive toward a partner. It's always a good idea to step back and think about how you are treated in a relationship, and how you are treating your partner in a relationship. If you recognize any of these symptoms in your relationship, you might want to think about talking to someone such as a hotline support staff member, health-care provider, counselor, or religious leader about what is hap-pening and get some support. If it feels scary, then it is wrong.

What You Can Do If It Happens to You

When a person is in an abusive relationship, it can be hard to ask for any type of help or support. A person may feel embarrassed, afraid, or unsure about where to go or what will happen next. People who are in abusive relationships may think that they should be able to "tough it out" or even fight back. It's possible a per-son may simply believe that control and force are a part of all relationships, even though this is not true. The person experiencing the abuse may love the partner. Relationships often don't start out being abusive; they start out exciting, with butterflies and nervousness like any other relationship. When someone starts to experience abuse, that person may hope the partner will go back to the way things were before the violence started. Or the abusive partner may be very loving and kind sometimes, and these times serve to reinforce the control and violence, and make it difficult to leave. For all these reasons, getting out of an abusive relation-ship may not be easy. It often takes courage, support, and knowing what to do. If you are in an abusive relationship and want to leave your partner, here are some strategies you might want to use:

Does *Twilight* Glamorize Violence in Relationships?

The *Twilight* series—both the books and the movies—has been very popular, and many fantasize about having a romance like the one between Bella and Edward. But their relationship doesn't seem so healthy to me, as Edward does a lot to control Bella. For example:

- Edward controls Bella by preventing her from seeing Jacob and not letting her drive (he even disables her car!). In a healthy relationship, there is more trust between partners.
- Edward often blames Bella for his anger, saying he feels that way because he loves her so much that he wants to kill her! No one partner is responsible for another's violent feelings and tendencies.
- Edward watches Bella while she sleeps and is always waiting for her. Couples need to set boundaries and have alone time.
- As Bella and Edward become closer, Bella slowly loses her friendships and relationships with her family. This is an example of isolation—one of the major aspects of a violent relationship.

While it's fine to enjoy the series, it's not a good idea to see that relationship as a model for romance.

- Tell someone you trust about your situation and experiences. Talk to your friends, but also talk to an adult (or two) that you trust—someone from your family, school, or church you think will listen and believe you; someone from your local Domestic Violence and Sexual Assault support agency, if you have one in your area; someone you believe can help you get out of a relationship that is unsafe because that person is supportive and knows about local resources. Remember: Some good people to turn to, such as teachers and health-care providers, are also mandatory reporters. This means they have to report any abuse to authorities.

- Work out a safety plan. Have your trusted person or people help you. If you are afraid that your partner will get mad and try to look for you to get you back, think about who can help you stay safe. Maybe call or text someone if you are by yourself. Identify where you will go if you aren't feeling comfortable in your surroundings—maybe there is a coffee shop or library or some other public place where you can hang out for a while. Set some times to check in with a friend so that people know you are OK or if you need some help.
- Do not meet your ex-partner alone. No matter how nice your ex is being, no matter how sorry this person seems, this individual has proven to be controlling and manipulative. Your ex might do or say anything to get you back. Do not believe that person—believe in yourself and trust your gut you are doing the right thing.

What You Can Do If You Are Raped

If you are raped, the first thing to remember is that it's not your fault. A rape is never the fault of the victim. Never, never, never. Someone chose to rape you. That person is responsible for what happened. The next thing you might consider is whether you want to tell anyone what happened, and if so, identify whom you want to tell. This is not an easy decision; I hope you will think about telling someone what happened because after a traumatic event such as a rape, it is good to get help and support. You can talk to a friend, a trusted adult in your life, a health-care professional, or law enforcement. No one should deal with the trauma of rape alone. Just remember—if you are under eighteen, certain adults are required by law to take legal action such as telling other authorities or pressing charges against your perpetrator. It will be hard to talk about what happened, but it's important. However, it does take some people years to talk about their rape experiences. There is no one right way to do it.

The Exam

Some people want to report their rapes and press charges against their perpetrator. If you think you want to do this, it is a good idea to go to a hospital and get a SAFE (sexual assault forensic evidence) exam, or rape kit. Before going to get this done, please do not bathe, shower, or wash yourself. You will want to, but it's important to resist cleaning yourself. This is because there may be small pieces of the rapist's clothing (like threads) or some of the rapist's semen or blood on you that can be valuable evidence. Place your clothes in a paper bag or wrap them in newspaper, or just leave them alone. Do not place them in a plastic bag, as plastic

> **Remember Emergency Contraception!**
>
> ● If you are concerned about the possibility of a pregnancy, look up where you can get access to emergency contraception (you can find out at bedsider.org/where_to_get_it). The earlier you take emergency contraception, the more effective it is.

can destroy some evidence. Also, do not wash the clothes, as that will also get rid of evidence. The sooner a doctor examines you, the more chance there is of finding blood or semen on your body, or on your clothes, from the person who attacked you.

During a SAFE exam, a specially trained health-care professional will examine you. This person is often a SANE nurse, which stands for sexual assault nurse examiner. This examination may feel uncomfortable, but it's needed to collect any evidence on your body to help tell the story about what happened, and a specially trained person also needs to make sure that you are OK. However, it's important to know that you have the right to say no to any part of the exam that you do not want to do. You get to say yes or no every step of the way. The health-care professional will ask you about your sexual experiences and your overall health. This is not because you did something wrong, but because certain facts are needed to do the exam. Then the person will ask you about what happened during the rape. Even if you feel scared or ashamed, or anything else, try to remember as many details as possible. You can have a friend, a parent, an advocate, or a counselor in the room with you if you like. Just ask for support if you want someone there with you. You do not have to be alone through any of this. Some hospitals have

Support for Survivors

SART stands for sexual assault response team. This is a group of people from the community that can coordinate a supportive response for a person who has experienced a sexual assault. This team may consist of health-care professionals such as a SANE nurse, a community-trained advocate, law enforcement, legal representative, judge, and/or other professionals who have the interest and desire to help those who have experienced sexual violence.

advocates on call who are trained to stay with you during this difficult time. You also have the right to ask anyone to leave the room that you don't want there.

The physical examination may also be difficult. The examiner will check your body for semen, bruising, cuts, and other injuries. This is not only to collect evidence, but also to make sure you are OK. Your pubic hair might be combed, and your whole body will be checked for cuts and bruises. If you scratched or bit the rapist, tell the examiner. She will scrape under your fingernails and document any harm that you may have done to the rapist while protecting yourself (more evidence). You will be offered an STD check and maybe emergency contraception. If you aren't offered emergency contraception and want some, ask for some yourself or ask your advocate to do it for you. Two weeks later, you should go to your regular doctor or clinic to get tested for STDs, including HIV. You want to be safe and make sure that you did not get any STDs during the assault.

Taking Legal Action

At some point, you might be able to decide if you want to press charges. If you do not want to, that is OK. You can still go through the medical examination, but if police are there, you can tell them that you do not want to press charges; they may still need to, depending on the circumstances. They still need to report and record the rape, so the police will put it in a casebook. They also will take the collected evidence, and you will be given a number referring to the evidence. If you do want to press charges, you can do so at any time, but know that in some states evidence is only kept for six months so time can be an issue. Ask an officer about your rights; an advocate or hotline might also know more about your rights based on where you live and how old you are.

Whatever you decide to do takes strength and courage. Many people benefit when someone decides to report because it helps others fight, and possibly makes them feel better as they seek justice. However, the process isn't easy. Many of you may have heard about the anguish of prosecuting a rapist. Many may have heard that a person should not bother pressing charges against a rapist because the person is just going to go free anyway. While there is unfortunately some truth to these statements, you should know that the laws and punishments against rapists are getting tougher these days.

Rapes are the most underreported crimes. That means that more rapes go unreported than any other crime in America. It is estimated that two-thirds of all rapes are not reported to the police.[5] There are many reasons that rapes are not reported. Survivors:

- Do not want to talk about what happened to anyone
- Fear that they will not be believed

Sports Take a Stand against Sexual Violence

In 2014, Major League Baseball and the National Football League up-dated policies against domestic violence. The leagues can now suspend players if they are charged with, or accused of (not just found guilty of), violence against their partners. The NFL also provides counseling and services for victims, families, and the accused.

- Do not want to go through the emotional trauma of the trial, even if their rapists are punished
- Fear that their rapists will hurt them further if they say what happened
- Know the rapist and do not want to get that person in trouble

All of these reasons make sense to some and do not make sense to others at the same time. These reasons may both make sense and not make sense in the same person. Some people may think that a crime should be reported, no matter what. Others may feel that the legal system cannot be trusted, and therefore they don't see why it makes any sense to report a rape. The reality is that criminal cases can last a long time, and sexual violence cases sometimes focus on and blame the survivor for the violence, and advocate for the perpetrators. This can be really hard and daunting to go up against. The bottom line is it's up to the person who was raped to make as many choices as the law will allow. If someone decides to press charges, that person should get support from the legal system, friends, and family.

Recovery Takes Time

Getting out of an abusive relationship and surviving sexual violence are not easy. But you can heal from the emotional trauma and stress that most people get from these experiences. The trick is, it's going to take a lot of help and support from others and hard work on your part.

Experiencing trauma has a big effect on both your body and your brain. When experiencing trauma, such as an abusive relationship or a sexual assault, your body goes into survival mode: certain parts shut down and other parts, like the stress response, go into high gear. Your blood pressure might go up; you might feel sick to your stomach; it's common to feel shaky. All of these symptoms are reactions to trauma. When experiencing high trauma and stress, a body can automatically go into fight, flight, or freeze mode. This means that when people experience sexual violence they may run away, fight back, or do nothing—the brain decides on its own. A person doesn't always have control over what the brain does during and in response to violence.

Trauma's long-term effects on the brain are equally, if not more, powerful than the short-term ones. After a trauma, people can feel a complete loss of control. They might feel the same short-term physical symptoms for a long time—not just right after the event, but also several days, weeks, or even months later. People might not trust themselves anymore and feel unsafe everywhere they go. People who experience sexual or dating violence can experience a lot of anxiety and uncertainty about the world and relationships. After trauma, a person may have a huge range of emotions—sadness, anxiety, anger, loneliness. It might even be hard to concentrate. Experiencing a trauma can completely change how a person sees the world.

While all of this impact that trauma has on the body and brain is very intense, it is perfectly normal. And the more intense the trauma is, or the more often it is experienced, the stronger the impact. Knowing all of this, if you have experienced trauma, it is important to seek help and support on your road to recovery. Talking to trusted and trained adults can be helpful. Mental health professionals

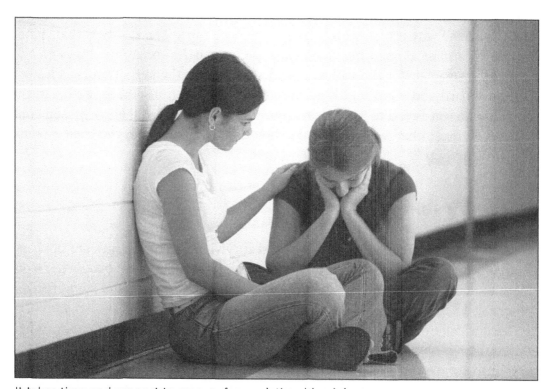

It takes time and support to recover from relationship violence.

who are experts in assisting people as they get through trauma may give you certain thought exercises to help you reprogram your brain into healthy, calmer ways of thinking. People in your support network—friends, family, clergy, or other community members—can check in on you to see if you are practicing self-care. Self-care is treating yourself with kindness, in the way you deserve to be treated. Eating healthy foods, getting plenty of rest, doing things that you enjoy, exercising, and meditating are all ways people can practice self-care. Surround yourself with people who see how beautiful you are. Love yourself. Give yourself time to heal.

Remember, you are never to blame for what happened. Show compassion for yourself, and understand that what happened was not your fault. In time, you will be stronger. Give yourself time to move past the experiences you had. Try not to compare yourself to others even though it's hard not to—think more about how everyone heals at the pace that is best for a specific situation and individual, and that there is no best way to recover. Talk to a counselor, or see if there are support groups in your area. Look for support groups online if you are in a rural area, or if you do not feel comfortable enough to talk about what happened in person. But in order to completely recover, most people need to talk to a professional eventually. Know that some days will be harder to face than others. That's OK. Bad days may be triggered by something that reminds you of your past abusive relationship or by entering a new one too fast. Talk to a counselor or

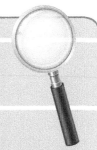

What You Can Do If a Friend Has Experienced Abuse or Rape

- Believe your friend's words and feelings.
- Be patient. It may take your friend a long time to recover from this event. Be there when you can, and as the difficult feelings come and go.
- Listen to your friend share what feels comfortable.
- Understand that it's ultimately your friend's choice as to whether to get help or report what is happening. Support your friend in whatever that person chooses to do.
- Get support for yourself if you are scared, feeling alone, or angry because of what happened to your friend (calling a hotline or talking to a counselor might help).

support group about these times and your feelings. Don't try to get through this by yourself. In time—sometimes a long time—you will be able to have a happy, healthy life either by yourself or with a special someone who treats you with the respect that you have always deserved.

Resources

The following websites are great resources for anyone who is in a violent relationship, or has been raped, and needs support. You can use them for yourself or a friend who wants help:

- Love Is Respect has a phone number, chat, and text line open all the time—24/7/365. Call 1-866-331-9474, chat at LoveIsRespect.org or text "loveis" to 22522.
- Rape, Abuse and Incest National Network (www.rainn.org) has a ton of information and resources to get help or find out how to support someone in need.

Not near a computer or don't have a data plan? Call the National Sexual Assault Hotline. It automatically directs you to the nearest sexual assault service provider: 1-800-656-HOPE (4673).

ANALYZING
INFLUENCES

••

If you have read this book up to here, you now know all the safer sex methods that are available to you. To recap, they are:

1. Choosing not to have sex (being abstinent)
2. Using a condom with a partner
3. Being monogamous, getting tested for sexually transmitted diseases (getting treated as necessary), and using birth control in order to avoid an unwanted pregnancy (if necessary)

You also have read about consent—what it is, why it's necessary, how to listen for it, and how to give it. Congratulations! You now know all there is to know about being sexually healthy—or do you? How many of you know someone who knows how to be safe and wants to be safe, but for some reason is not being safe when it comes to sex? There are a lot of people out there who "know better," but still end up in less-than-ideal sexual situations. This is because we live in a world that has many different influences on us and our peers when it comes to making sexual decisions. Our friends, partners, the media, and even our gender can all influence the ways we think about sex, and as a result, influence decisions about sex. Although there is no way one book can discuss all these influences in detail, it is worthwhile to take a look at them and think about how they might affect your life.

Peer Pressure Coming from inside You

Most of us hear about peer pressure from our parents and health teachers. We learn that we should not bend under peer pressure, that we should just say no, and that if our friends pressure us into doing something, then they are really not our friends. I think most of us can agree with those statements. I also think many of you would, rightfully so, defend your friends and say that your friends would never force you to do anything that you did not want to do. You can probably choose better friends than that. So does that mean that we aren't influenced by our friends and peers? Nope. We are all shaped by those we hang out with and what they think. This is because it's natural to do so. It feels good to agree with people, feel like we belong to a group, and generally get along with others. This is why the strongest type of "peer" pressure, oddly enough, exists in your own mind. What do I mean by that? Here are a few examples:

- You are hanging out with your friends who are all exchanging stories about their partners. They talk about what a good kisser this one is and how this guy really knows what to do "down there." Everyone is listening, asking questions, giggling, and having a good time. Meanwhile, you get very quiet. You have never been with anyone sexually. You are suddenly convinced that the whole party is going to turn to you and ask you what you think about all of this. You feel like you're missing out on something big, and start to feel left out because you believe you are the only person in the whole world who at sixteen has never hooked up with anyone . . .
- You are in the locker room after a game. The rest of the gang is talking about who they have "done" and bragging about their sexual exploits. You and your partner have talked about sex, but have decided to wait until you have been dating longer, or you want to wait until summer to have sex, when things are less stressful. You care about each other and are happy with the decision. Yet you find yourself telling the team that you have had sex and are even giving a few details about things that have never happened . . .
- You are texting your friend during sex ed class. For this particular lesson, your teacher talks about how sexually transmitted diseases can be transmitted via oral sex. Your friend texts, "Oral sex? Gross. Who would want 2 do that?" The truth is, you have, and you and your partner have enjoyed giving each other oral sex safely and responsibly. But now, for some reason, you feel ashamed about what you do and make a promise to yourself that you will never do it again . . .

All of these situations are ways your friends are influencing you, but they are not influencing you directly. They are not exactly telling you what to do and not do, but they are making you feel as though you are doing something wrong when it comes to sex. This is the way peer pressure often works. Friends usually aren't going up to you and saying what you should or should not do when it comes to sex. Instead, indirectly, your friends make you feel left out, or as though you are doing something wrong. It's completely normal to want to fit in, to want to contribute to a conversation. It's natural to want to be liked, or at least agree with what your friends are saying, especially if they are talking in a large group. If you feel close to someone, you might want to go along with what that person is say-

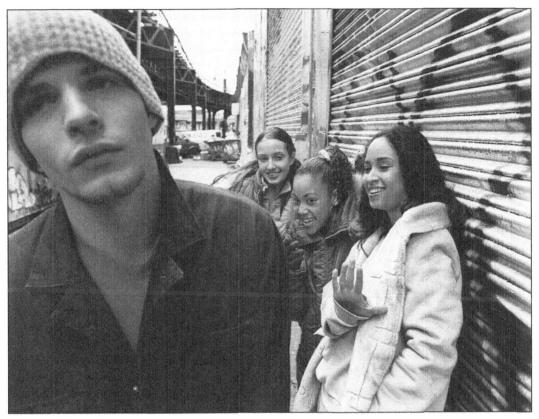

When it comes to sexual experience, it's easy to feel left out.

ing so you can feel even closer. It's understandable that you would listen to your friends to hear what are right and wrong things to do in a sexual situation. When what you do does not match what people are talking about, it's logical that you may worry—worry that you are the only person in the world who has or has not done a particular sexual act.

The thing to remember, however, is that sexual experiences are very personal. There is no timeline for when you should or should not do things. And, above all, it's not a race to see who can be the most sexually active first. Guinea pigs have sex for the first time when they are only a few days old. Does that mean that guinea pigs are the pimp-daddy, bad-ass animals of the kingdom? Does that mean that a three-day-old guinea pig is mature? Of course not. On the other end of the spectrum, lions, the kings and queens of the jungle, wait several years before having sex—are they an immature species? And gibbons stay with one partner for their entire lives—are they whipped? Hardly.

Now, I don't want to spend too much time comparing your sexual decisions to those of animals, but the point is, your decisions about your sexuality are exactly that—yours. The right decision and the wrong decision are not based on what your friends think—it's up to what you and your partner think. Your friends are not the ones who are involved in your sex life, and they can't tell you what will and won't fit into your life or make you feel good. Friends can give advice, and you can learn from your friends, but in the end it's up to you and your partner to figure out what you do and don't want to do sexually. It's hard not to care about fitting in, about doing "the right thing" according to your besties, but try to take a step back and think—if I have sex, if I decide not to have oral sex, or whatever, why am I deciding this? Is it for me, or is it so that I can feel more included or "normal"? If your reason for doing something sexual has anything to do with what your friends are doing or with acceptance, you may want to hold off on your decision a little longer.

Partner Pressure = No Consent

It is never OK to pressure your partner to do something your partner does not want to do sexually. If your partner says no to something, or in some other way does not give consent, it is not OK to ask again, whine, pout, get mad, or do anything else to pressure your partner (see chapter 8 for more about consent). It is always OK to say no to something you do not want to do sexually, even if you have done it before with the same or a different person.

Along the same lines, if you are not ready to have sex or want to stop a certain sexual activity you've done before with each other, talk to your partner about it. Choose a time when the two of you can sit down and talk together, face-to-face. Ideally, you can find a time before things get all sexy and romantic. Have this talk when the lights and your clothes are on, when the two of you can have a serious, undistracted conversation about what you do and do not want. If your partner isn't interested in having a conversation like this, that's a sign that your partner doesn't respect you or isn't ready to talk about sex (which means your partner, in my opinion, isn't ready to have sex). If someone does not respect you and your choices, that sort of relationship will go nowhere.

Once the two of you sit down and really hash it out, you may be surprised to learn that you and your partner are feeling the same way—your partner may not want to rush your sexual relationship any faster than you do; your partner may want to try something neither of you have done before. But you won't really know that unless you ask.

Just remember—if your partner forces you to have sex either through physical or emotional pressure, no matter how many times you have had sex before, that person is attempting or committing rape. And, in the same way, if you try to influence someone into doing something sexual with you when that person has not given consent, you are committing sexual assault. Having sex without consent is never acceptable.

Media Blitz: Sex on TV, in Music, and Online

It's true—there is a lot of sex in the media. Advertising agencies live by the motto "sex sells," talk shows lure us in with the not-so-secret tales of other people's sex lives, TV dramas are full of romance and betrayal, and sitcoms make sexual jokes all the time. Reality TV makes us think that we can "win" a partner through some kind of competition that's supposed to lead to true love. Popular songs and the videos that go along with them are full of sexual references—some pretty darn blunt. Online we can look up any sexual act one can imagine, and many you never knew existed but might stumble upon anyway through searching for information. But does being exposed to all of these sexual messages influence people in any way? Maybe they do some good—by exposing people to sex, perhaps the media is doing us all a favor by normalizing a behavior that many are too embarrassed to talk about in public. Or maybe all these media sources send inaccurate messages about how sex should and shouldn't be. There are as many opinions about sex in the media as there are people.

One fact is that people are exposed to a lot of sex thanks to the media. It's estimated that the average young person will see fourteen thousand sexual references in the media every year,[1] and each of these references has its own message about sex: That it's cool. Or dangerous. Or desirable. Or that only beautiful people have it. Or that only young people are sexual/sexy. Maybe the message is that it's spontaneous, or that it happens naturally. The bottom line is all media carries a message, and it's up to each of us to try to figure out what that message is—and how closely it resembles the truth about what sex really is and how it happens between two people. For example, out of all the TV programs that contain sexual content, only one out of seven mentions anything about STDs (sexually transmitted diseases) or planned pregnancy.[2] How realistic is that? How responsible is that?

The other thing that is weird about sex on television is that there is a lot of kissing and a lot of sex, but little else. Television shows people passionately kissing, and then, oftentimes, people have sex. There is no intimate touching, no "foreplay"—just straight from kissing to sex. Only 1 percent of the sex scenes on television show the couples having any sexual patience.[3] That is, once they started getting undressed, they were going all the way.

So here are the messages television tends to send when it comes to sex: that it's expected that romantic relationships include sex, without talking about the risks and responsibilities, and without engaging in any types of intimate touching or togetherness other than kissing. Another message is that once you start taking your clothes off, it means that you are going to have sex. And that's not really how things work in real relationships.

What Do *You* Think?

Some people say that shows like MTV's *16 and Pregnant* (2009–present), which follows teenagers through their pregnancies and childbirth, glamorize young parenthood. However, research published in 2014 found that the show may actually have led to *fewer* teen pregnancies! For example, after an episode aired, researchers noted that there were an increased number of Internet searches on birth control, and many young people tweeted reminders to themselves and others to take their birth control pills. It was estimated that teen birthrates fell by almost 6 percent in just a year and a half as a result of this show.[a]

Sex Online

There's a lot of sexually explicit content online, and just like there are different kinds of movies out there, there are different kinds of pornography. At the movie theater, there are blockbusters, independent films, comedies, dramas, and many other choices. Likewise, there's big-budget pornography, independent releases, feminist porn—all designed to appeal to different audiences (usually male audiences). And although it's illegal for people under eighteen years old to view it, younger people still view depictions of sex online—sometimes on purpose, sometimes not.

Making it illegal for anyone under eighteen to view pornography does two things: it can make it more desirable for a younger person to watch it, and it makes pornography seem like a very "dirty" and bad thing. There is some truth to the fact that viewing pornography can be harmful: not all porn is created equal; there are levels of intensity when it comes to porn, and these levels have a lot to do with how they potentially influence the behaviors of those who use it. When the sex is depicted using violent images like rape, forced sex, or bondage, studies have shown that this can make people more violent in their own relationships and lives in general.

One of the most important things to consider about watching sex online is that it is a form of adult entertainment. In other words, the sex a person sees does not reflect real sex, nor does it try to. In fact, it tries to do just the opposite. Sex online is a form of sexual fantasy, not an educational tool. The people who perform the sex acts are actors. Even the "amateur" videos contain actors, since those people are performing for an audience, in front of a camera.

If sex in real life were like sex online, here is what would and would not happen:

- Sex would last for hours and hours.
- No erections would be lost.
- Everyone would have a perfect body.
- No one would ask for consent before doing anything sexual.
- No one would check in with a partner to see if both people were enjoying it.
- Body hair would not exist.
- People would always moan and make lots of noise.
- There would be no need to discuss condoms, never mind use them.
- No one would get pregnant or contract an STD.
- No one would talk about feelings or emotions.
- Everyone's hair (and makeup) would look perfect when they were done having sex.

Very little is real about sex online, which is why it's not a good idea to learn about how to be sexual with another person by watching sexually explicit videos. A lot of the sexual behaviors you might see are more about fantasy sex than real sex, so don't think what you see is what you should do. As always, it's important to talk to your partner before doing any sexual behavior to see what the two of you both want to do.

Pornography: The Good and the Not-So-Good

Porn can both help and hinder a person's sexual health. Some ways that porn can benefit people:

1. It can help them fantasize about what they might like or not like.
2. It can be a safe visual aid for when people masturbate.

However, there are ways in which porn can harm a person's sexual health:

1. It can interfere with that person's desire to have a real relationship. Some people begin to depend on pornography in order to get sexual release.
2. It can create expectations that real-life sex is actually like the sex in videos. Video sex is exaggerated, as are the reactions of the people (they are acting, remember!). Real-life sex rarely lasts as long or is as exciting and "all that" as it appears online.

3. All the bad and messy parts about sex are magically missing from porn. No one ever loses an erection, gets a headache, or makes a funny noise.
4. It looks as though porn stars are always in the mood for sex. No one, I mean no one, is always in the mood for sex. Don't expect that attitude from your partner or yourself. Get and give consent!
5. It can make it seem as though, during sex, someone always needs to dominate another; that's not true. Sex between two equal partners can be an amazing experience.
6. It can cause people to have unrealistic expectations about what they and others look like naked. Breasts, penises, and other sexual body parts are not as big on most people as they are on the people in the videos.
7. In pornography, safer sex is rarely mentioned. Where are the condoms and the concerns about pregnancy and STDs? Get real!

The answer to the question many of you have—"Is it OK to like porn?"—cannot be answered in a book. It has to be answered by you. Whether you want to make pornography a part of your life is a decision only you can make (mind you, it is illegal for stores to sell porn to anyone under eighteen years old). Some people like all types of pornography, some people do not like any form of pornography. Some people are OK with certain types or various levels of intensity. The bottom line is, do what you feel comfortable doing, and make sure anyone else involved is comfortable, too.

The Influence of Gender Roles

Gender roles are how society thinks a person should act based on whether it sees that person as a man or a woman. As stated in chapter 2, there are more genders than simply these two, but when it comes to gender roles, the world tends to focus on just these two.

Gender roles are everywhere and are ever present. They happen as soon as a baby is born. Based on anatomy (is there a penis or vulva down there?), a baby is often dressed in blue or pink and then given toys that reflect the "proper" gender—dolls are given to girls, and trucks to boys. As children get older, those gender roles continue and creep into hobbies. Sure, some hobbies might be seen as OK for any gender, but there are still stereotypes at play here. For example, anyone can be interested in music, but what about the assumptions of who should play a flute versus a tuba? When it comes to sports, does it matter who tries out for the football team or the gymnastics team? Sadly, gender roles can determine whether people decide to pursue something that interests them, because they don't want to act outside of their gender role.

There are also strong gender roles when it comes to sexual activity and relationships, and we often play into them without thinking. For example, society perceives sexually experienced young men more positively than sexually experienced young women. These men are seen as being "studs" or part of the cooler crowd, while these women can be seen as "sluts" or "easy." On the other hand, young men who have less sexual experience are not always seen in a positive light, being thought of as "weak" or somewhat of a loser. Young women who are seen as being less sexually experienced are sort of stuck in a weird spot—they are perceived both negatively and positively. A young woman who chooses not to have sex might be considered a responsible person and at the same time a prude. But even being called responsible may not always seem so pleasant —it depends on who says it. If a parent says their child is responsible, or a "good girl," that is seen as praise and approval. But if someone in class rolls their eyes and says, "Anna? Hmph. She is such a *good* girl," the label takes on a completely different meaning.

What is pretty clear here is that this situation is hardly fair. The gender role for females pretty much shows that no matter what young women do, have sex or not have sex, they can be called some pretty hurtful things. And here is something else to think about—does a woman even have to have sex in order to be called a slut or whore? Nope. She might just wear some sexy clothing, show off a sense of confidence, and she could be considered "too sexual." Not natural, not normal, but worthy of negative names. Judging or belittling a young female for expressing her sexuality through her dress or actions is known as "slut shaming." The idea behind it is that young women should be limited in their sexual expressions in ways that young men don't need to be.

Meanwhile, the young men seem to at least have a plan of action if they are to avoid being perceived negatively. If they are sexual, they are perceived more positively (even players get a better reputation than losers). But what young men can't do is freely choose between two options. With young women, even though they might be perceived negatively whether or not they choose to have sex, at least they can choose. With young men, their choices are taken away from them. Have sex, or put yourself at risk for being subjected to negative labels.

That's not the only reason young men can't win by buying into gender roles. Not only do men lose their choices about what they can and cannot do, but the ways in which they can "earn" a more positive label are not the greatest ideas, to say the least. Think about it. In order for a guy to earn a reputation as *the man*, what else can he do besides have sex? Well, he can:

- Fight
- Drink alcohol or use drugs (the more the better)
- Carry a gun
- Accept a challenge (like jumping off a high place, or racing his car)

Most of the things you need to do to earn such a title are downright dangerous. They could cost you your health, or even your life. Why risk your liver, brain, or life simply to be known as someone who parties a lot or gets plenty of action?

And simply doing these sorts of things is not even enough. Someone buying into this male gender role has to *win*. He needs to be better than the next guy. If he fights and loses, he is no longer *the man*, he is *loser*. And if he has sex one weekend, his conversation with friends might look like this:

> *Guy 1:* Hey—did you get some this weekend?
> *Guy 2:* Yeah, you bet.
> *Guy 1:* Awright dawg!!

But then next week, this happens:

> *Guy 1:* Hey—did you get some this weekend?
> *Guy 2:* Naw.
> *Guy 1:* What happened?

Why should you have to explain yourself just because you had sex one week, but not the next? Or here is another scenario:

> *Guy 1:* Hey Michael! Have you been gettin' any lately?
> *Guy 2:* Boy, did I ever get some good lovin' last week. Feels nice just thinking about it.
> *Guy 1:* Last week?!?!? I had sex three times just yesterday!

What these situations show is that if you work hard to fit into the ideal male gender role, you will end up "losing" because there is always someone "better" than you—getting more dates, having more sex. Why bother entering a race you can't win? Besides—there are some things in life where quality is more important than quantity, and sex is certainly one of those.

> *Question:*
> Are girls equally sexually active as boys are? It's said that a girl's sexual excitement is eighteen times more than that of a boy.
> —Nineteen-year-old

> *Answer:*
> Girls can certainly be as sexually active as the boys and are sometimes more interested in sex than their male peers.

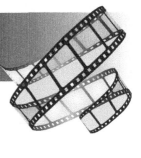

Movie Review: Easy A (2010, 1h 32m)

A high school student (Emma Stone) lies about losing her virginity and earns a reputation of being the class slut without ever having kissed anyone before.

When it comes to sexual excitement or interest in sex this is very individual across genders and it is difficult to make generalizations. Many people feel adolescent boys are more active sexually than the girls because they are more encouraged by the culture to be active and in general have more freedom from parental control.

Hope this helps,

Health Professional, We Are Talking, teen health website[4]

Women in Music

Though girls and women who express themselves as sexual beings are often called sluts, the one place where it's cool to be a slut—or at least a tease— seems to be in music. Madonna, in her early days, totally redefined female sex and sexuality with her crazy cone-bra outfits and songs "Like a Virgin" ("touched for the very first time") and "Papa Don't Preach" ("I'm keeping my baby"). Now artists like Beyoncé, Lady Gaga, Katy Perry, and Rihanna are seen as both sexy and powerful performers.

However, sometimes sex appeal in music seems to be equated with how little the performer wears or her dance moves. Think about the uproar Miley Cyrus caused when she twerked with Robin Thicke at the 2013 MTV Video Music Awards. And let's not forget when Janet Jackson (the "Nasty Girl") exposed her nipple during her "wardrobe malfunction" at the 2004 Super Bowl halftime show.

How the Heck Do I Think Differently from Everyone Else?

So what can each of you do to stop stereotyping people who are and are not sexually active? How can you shake the gender roles that put people in undesirable and unhealthy places? I am sure you can think of some ways on your own, but to give you a head start, here is a short list:

1. Stop thinking that there are only two genders! Once you open up your world to the idea that there are many different genders, it's easier to open up to the idea that there are many ways people act sexually, and they can all be considered "normal."

2. Recognize that you live in a world of stereotypes. By just recognizing the names we call people who do and do not have sex, you are well on your way to thinking about people in a more inclusive manner. Thinking criti-

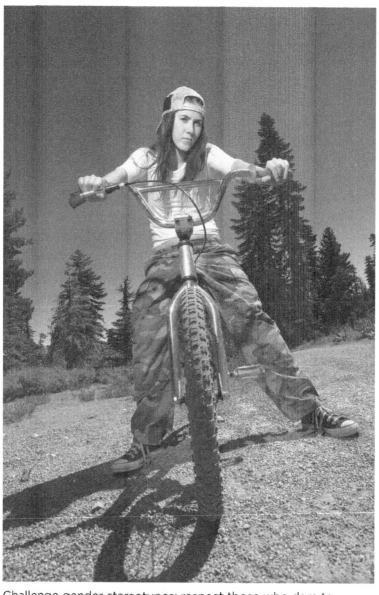

Challenge gender stereotypes; respect those who dare to.

cally about these names is one way to fight and challenge the stereotypes that surround you.

3. Think about each person as an individual. Each person has his or her own reasons for doing things. Every person and situation is unique. Remember that, and it becomes harder to label people based on their actions or reputation.

4. Put yourself in another person's place. Next time you think of someone as a player, or slut, or loser, think about why you jump to that conclusion. What do you really know about this person? Are the rumors you hear true? And if they are, does that person really deserve that name?

There is another really good reason to stop believing in these gender roles. The more you believe in slut shaming, make fun of people who choose not to have sex, and pump up young men for being sexually active, the more you will believe that's how the world should be. And if you believe in this way of the world, you might pressure yourself into playing into a gender role. So, if you are a young

It's Not Just Gender

When it comes to sexual stereotypes, gender is only one of the characteristics society makes assumptions about. In general, assumptions are made about the sexual attitudes and behaviors of people of different:

- Races
- Ethnicities
- Abilities
- Sexual orientations
- Gender identities
- Ages
- Appearances

Think about the assumptions and stereotypes given to these different groups of people. Know that they aren't accurate. A person's sexuality and sexual desires are unique and more complicated than a stereotype.

woman, and you think that young women who express their sexuality or have sex are sluts, then when you feel sexy, you may think of yourself as a slut. As a result, instead of feeling good about yourself, you might feel ashamed. In the same way, if you are a young man and for whatever reason you do not want to have sex one day, you might think something is the matter with you because if you truly were a stud, you would not give up the chance to "get some." Believing in these gender roles can only hurt you and those around you.

SEX AND RELATIONSHIPS ONLINE AND ON YOUR PHONE

Texts, social networks, private messages, apps, video games, and even emails and digital worlds are just some of the things you can use to communicate with another person without being face-to-face. And if you can communicate with someone digitally, you can flirt and develop relationships with people digitally. For the most part, digital interactions are a great way to meet people and help support and grow existing relationships. Having part of a relationship exist in the digital world is normal; we all interact in a world where we reach out to people in numerous ways, depending on the situation. In fact, having a separate section on digital communication might even seem a little odd, given that face-to-face communication and other forms of interaction are so interconnected. However, there are some specific things to consider when it comes to digital communication as you develop relationships with other people.

Digital Communication

There are many reasons to communicate with someone digitally rather than face-to-face. First of all, it's easier; the two of you may not live close together or even go to the same school, so meeting in person becomes difficult. Second, sometimes it's more practical; there are times when spending time together in person is simply not possible. Third, sometimes sending off a text is easier and more convenient than a phone call or face-to-face meeting. For example, making plans for Saturday night is sometimes best done with text or group messaging.

Then there are other, more complicated reasons for communicating with a partner on your phone or computer. Sometimes it's easier to meet someone or start a relationship indirectly on social media. Maybe you find someone you think is interesting who's a friend of a friend on social media, and you start connecting. Or maybe you meet someone at a party or in class, exchange phone numbers, and the two of you get to know each other better through texting or private messaging. Other times, couples message each other because they don't get the chance to spend a lot of time face-to-face because of busy schedules. Whatever the reason, different forms of online communication can help a relationship grow and bring people closer together.

Sometimes people who are already in a relationship believe it's easier to talk about certain things this way. It might be easier for you to say things to your partner online than it is to say them face-to-face. When you express how you feel to another person, you are taking a big risk, and sometimes not having to look your partner in the eye makes it easier to say things. You don't have to worry as much about immediate rejection, or some other negative reaction. Telling someone how you feel whether in person or through a text takes guts, no matter how you do it.

Simply put, communicating indirectly with a partner is a part of normal life. Therefore, it's important to think carefully about which parts of that relationship you want to keep public, and which parts you want to keep private in both the face-to-face and digital worlds. For example, if you and your partner go to the same school, you two together decide whether to hold hands or kiss in the hallway between classes—or perhaps you only show physical affection when the two

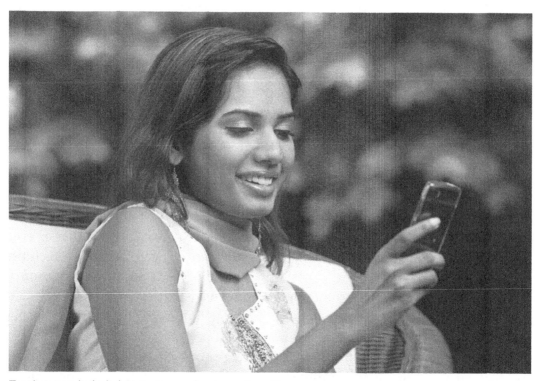

Texting can help bring two people closer together.

of you are alone. In the same way, you can choose to interact with your partner by sending notes through social media in a more public way (like on a wall or in a comments section) or in private (like through a text). There is one difference though. Whereas a kiss in private remains a kiss in private, a private message or

---

Youth Speak Out:
How Social Media Effects Relationships, by Olivia, Age 17

Social media can be a safe haven; a place where someone can vent about how tough life is, how annoying a co-worker is, or portray an alter-ego in a cyber society rather than in reality. Social media can also be a claim to bragging rights; a place to tell everyone about how much weight someone lost, how great their make-up looks, or how amazing their Hawaiian vacation is. It can be a perfect place for people to talk about just how wonderful their significant other is and how phenomenal it is to be with them. In other cases, social media can be a nightmare. The jealous one finds herself stuck at every turn. With the easy availability social media brings us, anyone can do thorough research on *that person* who likes too many of a partner's pictures on Instagram, retweets too many of their posts on Twitter, and constantly comments on their Facebook status updates.

For me it was the difficulty of watching someone I don't know have a great conversation with my boyfriend in the comments section of an Instagram post. I clicked, poked, and prodded through her profile to learn who she was, what she was doing, and why she was randomly talking to *my* boyfriend. With every dead end I found myself getting more and more frustrated. Upon bringing it up with my boyfriend, he got offended at my lack of trust and inability to calm down. But what else could he expect from me? Trust in a relationship is, at times, hard enough to come by. With the accessibility of getting to know someone else on the Internet, how could one not be constantly skeptical of what's really going on on the other side of their partner's screen?

Relationships can be hindered by situations like this. In my case, I broke up with my boyfriend and felt the glorious sensation of stress, jealousy, and frustration leave my body. Social media will always be around, so people have to find ways of coping with the feelings its presence may ignite, no matter how potentially detrimental to a relationship.[a]

picture can be made more public if one person forwards that message or shares it. It's important to figure out between the two of you what is private and what can be shared more publicly. If you don't know, and something was sent to you privately, you should consider it private until you ask your partner if it's OK to share it.

There are some downsides to digital communication, too. If couples rely too much on Internet and phone communication, they might lose the ability to talk to each other in person! Always think about balance: share things with your partner in both the online and face-to-face worlds. A mix of communication methods is often best for a healthy relationship.

Another negative feature of digital communication is that people sometimes think it's easier to say unkind things to each other through texts and in social media than in person. This is because, in some ways, the computer makes it less personal and puts distance between two people so that it is easier to make fun of someone or tell that person off. Please think about anything you post or type that is mean to another person. There is a live human being on the other end of your message. Before you hit Send, imagine saying what you typed right in front of that person. If you find that you can't do it, you probably shouldn't send it. In general, you shouldn't send unkind messages to anyone, no matter how justified you think you are. Messages like that are best given face-to-face—or not said at all. Think before you post or hit Send, because it's impossible to take something back once you do.

Finally, one of the positives of digital communication can turn into a negative if abused. The convenience of texting means that you can message your partner anytime, anywhere. While this can really help two people feel more connected to each other, sometimes it's hard to set boundaries between you and another person. It's possible to have too much contact with your partner in a relationship. For example, there may be trouble in the relationship if:

- One person texts the other all night (or you text each other back and forth) so that neither of you gets a good night's sleep
- One person constantly messages the other to see what's up, to the point where the partner feels uncomfortable
- Someone gets anxious if a partner doesn't respond to the message right away, and then questions that person about the delayed response when they see each other again—or keeps on texting until a response is given

These examples show that texting can be used to control the behavior of another person. No matter how it's done, controlling another person is never right. If you are uncomfortable with the way someone is communicating with you online or via text—whether it's happening too much or happening at times

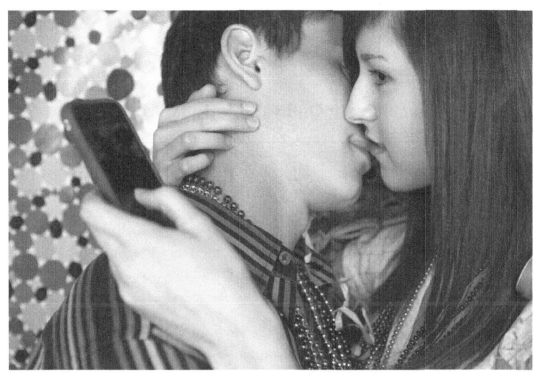

Don't let digital communication get in the way of quality face-to-face time with your partner.

that don't work for you—it's important to talk to that person and explain what is going on. Know what your limits are and try to communicate them. If a person doesn't pay attention to your boundaries and ignores your requests, that's a sign that the person doesn't respect or trust you—it may be time to end the relationship, or at least take a step back. In the same way, if someone talks to you about messaging too much or too late at night or during family dinner time, you need

Put the Phone Away at Night

One study found that over half of high school students texted after bedtime, and one in five were woken up because someone was texting them too late. This late-night texting behavior was associated with insomnia, feeling tired during the day, and worse grades in school.[b] The moral of this story is to say good night to your friends and partner, and tell them you'll talk tomorrow—your future depends on it!

to respect that person's time. After all, if you care enough to be in a relationship with someone, you should care enough to give that person the space needed to be the person you like so much.

Having an Exclusively Online Relationship

Sometimes it happens: two people who have never met face-to-face want to begin and maintain a romantic relationship online. Meeting people online has its good points: you can meet people that you otherwise would never run into, as geography no longer gets in the way. You can meet people with similar interests quite easily; all you have to do is go to an online community that talks about things that you like and bingo! People who have your same interests are right there along with you. So, those are the good points. Here are some things to consider about having a long-distance, completely digital, relationship:

- The person on the other side of the keyboard may be lying. Until you actually meet face-to-face, you honestly do not know who that person really is. Be careful about falling for someone you have never met face-to-face, as that person may or may not be telling you the truth.
- Online relationships tend to move a lot faster than relationships in real life. Why this is, I am not exactly sure, but I have some ideas. Part of the reason is that some people can spill their guts more easily on a keyboard than if they are looking someone in the eye: typing "I love you" can be a lot easier than saying it to someone. It can feel less risky. It also might be easier to say "I love you, too" when it simply is not true.
- It can be easy for each person in a digital relationship to fill in the blanks about the other person in ways that are perfect. Each person in the relationship can build up expectations, sometimes ones that are unrealistic, because it's easier to read between the lines online than deny the flaws of a person who is actually in front of you. You find your perfect match online because you can help create that person in your head.
- Be suspicious of those who want to know too much. Just as if you were meeting someone in person for the first time, there are certain things that are very personal that you would probably not talk about right away. People who ask personal details very soon should make you suspect their motivation for talking to you. Trust your instincts; if someone is making you feel uncomfortable, stop all communication.
- It's almost a contradiction, but also be wary of people who tell you practically nothing about themselves after the two of you have been chatting for a while (weeks, months). People who never want to talk about them-

selves are probably hiding something, like another relationship or the less-pleasant parts of themselves (hey—we all have faults, and those need to come out in any relationship).

- What is your level of commitment to someone you meet online? What is that person's commitment to you? If you have an online relationship with someone, is it OK to flirt with someone at your school? Can you go on a date with someone from your neighborhood? Can you have another online romance? Can you hook up with someone in person? People's feelings can get hurt if you do not talk about what is and is not OK. Talking about what an online relationship means and its boundaries is just as important as talking about the same things in a face-to-face relationship.
- It's really easy to be dumped online, so be careful about being hurt. Love is always risky, but it's even riskier online. It is very easy for people to simply stop texting and even change their number. They don't have to look you in the eye when they pull the plug on your relationship—they just have to message that it's over. If that happens, you are left alone with a lot of questions and no way to get them answered. People who do this are total cowards, but they're out there.

Meeting an Online Partner Face-to-Face

There are safety concerns when it comes to meeting people in person whom you first met online or just connected with on an app that tells you who's in your area or near your hangout spot. There are ways to keep yourself safe if you want to meet someone you've connected with on social media. First, don't give out personal information online such as your last name, phone number, where you live, or even your private email address. People can use this information to find you, and intentions might not be honorable. Second, no matter what's in a person's profile, you have to remember that a person may not be telling the whole truth or may be hiding something. This may be the case even if you chat and write to this person for months. Finally, if you do decide to meet someone in person you have only known online or just connected with on an app, meet that person in a public place. Ideally, you should bring a friend or two along. If this person really wants to meet you, that person will understand and respect your wishes to be safe. Encourage this new person to bring some friends along too, to make it a group meeting. If there is any objection, that is your cue to walk away. Also, let another friend or even your parents know where you are going. That way, if something happens, someone knows where you were last seen and who you were supposedly with. There is no reason to think this is overkill. Meeting someone in person you only knew through social networking is just like going on a blind date. As much as you would like to think otherwise, you might not really know who this person is and if that person deserves your trust.

Sexting: Being Intimate in a Digital World

Whether or not to sext, or send sexy pictures of yourself to another person, is a complicated issue. Some couples choose to do this to show how they feel about each other. If these pictures are kept private, most of the time there is no problem. If someone wants to send you a naked picture, that probably means the person trusts you very much and you should respect what that means to your relationship. If you are thinking of sending a naked picture of yourself to someone else, you need to think about your relationship with, and how much you really trust, that person. Only very special people deserve that level of trust from you. Overall, sexting can be a part of a healthy relationship, but it certainly isn't a necessary part. Just like other sexual behaviors, sexting may be something you and your partner choose to do or not; the important thing is that the two of you talk about it first to see if it's something you both would want to do and enjoy. Then, if sexting happens, it should be like any other sexual act: done responsibly, with consent, and maturely.

Reasons to sext:

- You want to.
- You want to send someone you care about a part of yourself.
- You want to express yourself sexually to someone you trust and care about.
- The person who will receive the text loves and cares about you and will enjoy it.
- You want to use it as a substitute for sex/safer sex because you want to wait/can't have sex for whatever reason.

Reasons not to sext:

- You don't want to.
- Someone is pressuring you to do so.
- You want to feel accepted.
- Someone is promising something in return for your picture.
- You are concerned about getting a bad reputation.
- You don't trust the person enough to keep the picture private.
- You're concerned about the legal consequences (in some states, it's illegal to send naked pictures of anyone—even yourself—if you are under eighteen years old).

Although there is a lot of talk about sexting in the media and possibly at your school, sexting, according to research, is pretty uncommon. Four percent of young people have sent a naked picture of themselves to another person, and young men and women are equally likely to send sexts. However, 15 percent of young people say they have received a naked picture of someone on their phone— that means that pictures that shouldn't be forwarded to others are anyway.[1] If you receive a sext—whether or not you asked for it—do not forward it to anyone else. It's important to respect people's privacy.

Even though young men and women report being equally likely to send a sext, young women are more likely to say they are distressed by doing it. This may be because young women are more likely to feel pressured into sending pictures of themselves, or may be more likely to do it in order to start a relationship, keep a relationship, or please a partner. It may be because they want to feel accepted by a guy or their peers. Yet, when they do send a sext after being pressured, sometimes they are seen as being insecure or having poor judgment. Also, there is still a double standard out there when it comes to women expressing their sexuality; while they are encouraged to do so, some are then considered slutty when they do! And if they don't send a picture, they are considered a prude. Young men do not feel this same pressure as often and sometimes are able to gain social status through sexts. Rarely do young women benefit the same way (see chapter 10 on how gender influences sexual pressure).[2]

Sexting should be in the context of give-and-take and not be one-sided; it doesn't seem right to have one person sending all the pictures. No matter who you are, never send someone a picture if you feel forced to do it, or in order to get someone to like you more or notice you. Sexting should be fun, not anxiety or guilt producing (sure, you might get jitters, but it should not feel shameful or wrong). In the same way, you should never ask someone else to send a naked picture as a dare, a joke, or just because you want to see what someone looks like without clothes. Sending pictures like this should only be done in the context of a relationship that's already pretty serious. Showing someone your naked body can be as intimate as having sex, and sexts should be treated with the respect and maturity that they deserve.

What to Do If You Receive a Sext

If someone sends you a sext, don't send it to anyone else. Period. If the sext was meant for you, then that's great: you were the proper recipient and it should not go beyond you; it violates the trust and respect of another to pass it on. If the sext you received wasn't a picture of the person who sent it to you, same thing: don't pass it on to anyone else. It wasn't meant for you, and that means it wasn't meant for others, either. And then, no matter whose image it is, delete it immediately. You don't want to have a nude image of someone else on your phone for many reasons. First, it can be disrespectful to keep it if it wasn't sent to you directly. Second, even if the image was meant for you, it could be illegal to keep it on your phone. This is because having a naked image of someone under eighteen years old could be considered being in possession of child pornography, and you certainly don't want to deal with that. Finally, some experts state that if you receive a sext, it is probably best *not* to tell an adult. I know in many cases turning to a trusted adult is a good thing to do, but this is an exception. This is because many trusted adults (for example, teachers) are either required or simply think it's a good idea to tell law enforcement about the image. That could lead to a lot of trouble for you and others.[3] So keep things simple and delete any sext as soon as you get it—no matter who sent it to you and for whatever purpose.

Cybersex

There are also times when a person sexts without pictures; this is sometimes called cybersex, or talking "dirty." Cybersex is when you type out the sexual behaviors you would like to do with someone and that person does the same back to you. Two (or more) people engage in cybersex either through texts or private messages. Having cybersex may not seem like such a big deal—after all, you can't get someone pregnant or get a sexually transmitted disease from it. But, after engaging in cybersex, some people feel strange about it. Sometimes cyber-sex can feel like the real thing—after all, it is an intimate activity where you are sharing feelings, ideas, and sexual fantasies. Afterward, people can feel closer to each other, may regret doing it, may not be sure if it means they now are in an in-person romantic relationship with someone, or may simply be confused about their emotions, and specifically their feelings toward sex and this person.

Know the Facts

- Private messaging apps like SnapChat seem like a safe way to send sexy photos because they disappear after they're viewed. However, it's important to know while these apps do add a layer of privacy and secrecy to your pictures, the receiver can take a screenshot of the phone, saving the picture that supposedly "went away"—and the app doesn't always let users know if this happens! Also, it's not such a great idea to send a picture to someone you don't know; pictures are for people you know and trust.

Revenge Porn

Revenge porn (also sometimes called sextortion) is sending out sexually explicit pictures or videos of another person without permission from that individual. These images may originally have been taken with or without consent. Sometimes, simply threatening to send the pictures or videos is considered revenge porn because the person with the pictures can threaten or blackmail someone into staying in a relationship or doing something else. Doing anything against someone's will—including engaging in revenge porn—is a form of sexual violence and more and more laws are being enacted to try to prevent it, or at least seek punishment for those who engage in it. As of 2016, states have laws against revenge porn.[c] Visit the Cyber Civil Rights Initiative at http://www.cybercivilrights.org for more resources if you have concerns about this issue.

My advice to you about cybersex is to treat it like real sex. If you do not know the person, do not have cybersex—in the same way that you would not have sex with someone you do not know in person. Only have cybersex with someone with whom you would have actual sex. So many people teach you to respect your body when it comes to sex; you should also respect your heart and your mind. Your heart and mind are just as involved—if not more involved—in sex as your body is. Therefore, seriously consider how you are going to think and feel after you have cybersex before you do it.

Getting Information and Support Online

Looking Up Information Online

While Internet pornography is not a great way to learn about sex (see chapter 10), there is great information about sex and sexual health on the Internet. However, searching for sex information online can be tricky. Here are some tips for finding the information you want—without being overwhelmed by images showing every kind of sex act imaginable (along with some you had never imagined).

First, try to get your search terms right and as specific as possible. Simply typing "sex" into a search engine is too broad, and will most likely not get you the accurate information you need. Try to be more specific about what you want to know. Make an effort to use formal medical terms for body parts you are curious about; add the word *education* to the end of your search term (for example, type "oral sex education" instead of just "oral sex"). Second, you might want to start your search on a medical site such as WebMD or the Mayo Clinic, or use one of the sites suggested in the resource section at the end of this book.

Once you find a site, you aren't done—you now need to figure out if the information you found is reliable! One way to do this is to use the ABCs method to size up a website to see if you should believe what it has to say:

- *A is for Author:* Who wrote what you're reading? Are you more likely to believe something a doctor wrote? A young person like yourself? A religious leader? Think about who is behind the words you are reading when you try to figure out how accurate the information is.
- *B is for Business Model:* Every website has to fund itself. How is the website you are on making its money? Is the site run by one person who is funding the project and doing all the work as a solo venture? Is the website trying to sell you something like a book to learn more, or a drug to enhance your sexual performance? Hint: Click on the "About Us" link on a website to find out who is behind it all!
- *C is for Current:* When was the article written? You want to make sure what you are reading is the latest information available. What we knew about sex in the early 2000s is a lot different from what we know today. Stay up to date to make the best decisions about your sexual health.
- *S is for Source:* Does the article you are reading tell you where the information came from? If a site makes a statement, does it say where that information came from? If someone makes huge claims about things, but doesn't back up those claims with research, you may want to think twice about believing what you read.

Finally, no matter how reliable online information seems, look at more than one site before drawing your own conclusions. There are a lot of facts and opinions out there—do your research and think critically before deciding what information deserves your attention.

Getting Support Online

For some people, online communities are a great place to learn about and explore a part of their sexuality that they aren't ready to talk about with someone in person. For example, some people who are thinking about their sexual or gender orientation feel that the Internet can be a great place to go to find a community where asking questions and meeting people can feel safe. Those living in a small town may be especially drawn to online communities, as there might not be a lot of resources locally for them to meet others they can relate to, or learn more about different forms of sexual attraction and expression. People of all sexual preferences and gender identities exist online, and many are happy to help guide someone who feels lonely or has questions. However, it's important to be careful and only participate in a community that is accepting and is honestly trying to help. If you are searching for an online community for your own sexual explorations, make sure that the people you are communicating with online are listening to you and aren't trying to change you. People you can trust will also not try to meet you privately. When young people are questioning who they are, they can be very vulnerable, and unfortunately, some people try to take advantage of that. Trust your gut if something doesn't feel right. If someone ever tries to force you to do something or frightens you in any way, it's OK to talk to a trusting adult about it or report that person using a website's Terms of Service (only the good ones will have something like this, so look for it!).

Also, it's important to not overlook the power of face-to-face communication. In one study in Australia, young people talked about the importance of face-to-face contact with other young lesbian, gay, bisexual, transgender, queer, and intersex people in a "safe" space. Even though half of the research participants stated that the Internet was a place where they could find friends they could trust, and three out of four said the Internet was a place where they felt accepted, they also mentioned how only interacting in online communities could make them feel isolated. These young people were able to create and maintain relationships that helped them explore their identities but, in the end, face-to-face contact could address this isolation in a way that online technologies could not.[4]

OTHER IMPORTANT TOPICS

••

I have learned many things as a sexuality education teacher, researcher, and online sex and relationship adviser. One of the most important things I have learned is that many young people have many questions about sex, sexuality, and relationships that are not usually covered in sex education books or classes.

Here, I talk about some of the more common, yet "secret" topics so that you can better understand some of them and also to let you know that they aren't strange or unimportant. Lots of people have questions about all of this stuff.

Talking with Parents and Other Adults about Sex

Talking with adults about sex and relationships can be a lot different from talking with them about other things. It can also be a lot different from talking to your friends or partner about sex. This is especially true if the adult in mind is a parent, or someone who is legally responsible for you. Each family is unique, so it makes sense that there is no one way that families talk about sex. Parents and caregivers across families allow for varying levels of discussion and disagreement from their children. You probably have a good idea of what you can and cannot say to a parent or caregiver. But, when in doubt, try opening up. You may be surprised with the results. And, if your parent or caregiver refuses to talk to you about sex, at least you know you tried.

Here are a couple of things to consider before talking with a parent or caregiver about something personal related to sex or relationships. First, one key to talking with caregivers about sex or relationships is to listen to what they have to say. True, you may feel as though your parent has no clue about what is going on in your life, or what things are like when it comes to romantic relationships or sex in people your age, but sometimes parents and caregivers are able to take a different perspective on a situation that might be useful—they might bring up things to consider that you haven't thought about before. Also, asking a parent or caregiver for advice and then listening to what they have to say might get you some respect, show them you can be mature, and allow you to understand where they are coming from. You do not have to agree with their point of view necessarily, but giving parents and caregivers the opportunity to talk may give you a better chance of being heard in return later on (bonus points).

If you disagree with a caregiver's expectations or wishes, talk about it. You may not "win" the argument, but expressing your opinion allows him or her to get to know you better and may help you be heard sometime in the future. Talk in a calm voice when everyone has plenty of time to hash out the problem areas. This also helps show that you are getting older, more responsible, and mature enough

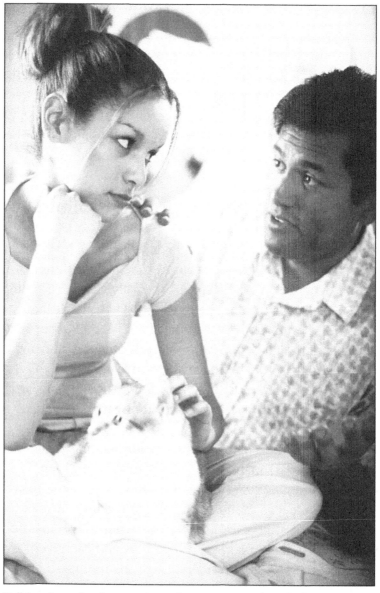

Talking to a family member about sex can be challenging, but also rewarding.

to handle tougher decisions and bigger issues. Whining and yelling doesn't make a good impression, and nothing much gets accomplished (except maybe a fight) if an intense conversation feels rushed.

Why It Might Be a Good Idea to Talk to a Parent, Caregiver, or Other Adult

There are times where something happens to you—like an unplanned pregnancy, a painful breakup, or a sexual assault—and it's better to deal with the problem with the support of others. While talking to a friend about what happened is a great idea, sometimes talking to an adult—especially a parent or legal guardian— is an even better idea. At first even the thought of talking to that person about serious personal issues may sound crazy, but think about it—parents and caregivers have some advantages:

- Like it or not, sometimes authority figures listen more closely to an older person. Getting an adult to represent you or stand beside you when you need to be official about something might make your side of the story more believable and seem more urgent.
- Many times, an adult who has been close to you a long time understands you in a way no one else can. While this isn't always the case, parents and caregivers more often than not step up to support their children the best way they can.
- A parent you have grown up with has known you your whole life, and may be able to understand you and what you are going through better than you think.
- Sometimes you need a parent or legal guardian to give you permission to do something, like get an abortion. You might need a parent's or legal guardian's OK to use health insurance to get an exam or birth control.
- Talking to your parent or caregiver about difficult issues might bring you closer together. At first there may be a lot of yelling and tension, but in the end, going through a rough time can bring people closer together.

There are situations and times when going to a parent is not a good idea or simply not possible. Your parent or guardian might be the cause of your situation or might have made it clear before that you cannot discuss certain circumstances, or you might not feel safe. In these cases, talking to another trusted adult or calling a hot line where adults have volunteered their time because they want to help young people in need can be a better option than going to a parent or caregiver who is not capable of giving you the support you need. Sometimes other adults

Youth Speak Out:
Talking to Your Parents about Sex, by Natalya

Do you feel like you're ready for sex but don't know whether or not to involve your parent(s)? When in a serious and/or sexual relationship, it may seem like a daunting task to approach your parents about your sex life. Even if some teens share a comfortable and open relationship with their parents, sex may not always be the topic of shared dialogue. While it can be nerve-racking at first, opening up and introducing a new level of honesty and trust between you and your parent(s) concerning sex can be an enlightening experience; your parent(s) may provide you with information regarding birth control, condoms, STDs, and even the emotional impact of sex that you'd never known before. Here are four simple tips to starting the conversation.

1. *Begin indirectly.* Jumping straight into a conversation about sex seems near impossible for those already dreading parental involvement. By first approaching parents with something that is related to sexuality (but not your sex life specifically), such as a new fact you learned about birth control or teen pregnancies, can help the conversation naturally progress. This familiarizes the topic of sex between the parents and the teen.

2. *Remind yourself about the purpose of the discussion.* Having trouble remembering why exactly you got yourself into this somewhat distress-inducing mess? No worries! Try and keep in mind that you facilitated this discussion because you are interested in being a healthy, responsible, sexually active teen. Remind yourself that your safety is of utmost importance, and you want to be as knowledgeable and honest about sex as you can.

3. *Ask your parent(s) about their teen/young adult sex lives.* If it's not too intrusive, ask about your parents' sex lives when they were your age (or perhaps a bit older). Doing so can allude to the fact that you are curious about sex. Additionally, bringing up your parents' pasts may make it easier for them to relate to or identify with you, transforming the dynamic of the conversation. Hearing stories from their past also carries the possibility of swaying or changing your opinion on being sexually active.

4. *Cut to the chase.* Be blunt, be honest, be open. Let your parents know that you've decided you want to become sexually active but also want to maintain a sense of trust and integrity between both parties. Communicate with your parents that safety is incredibly crucial to your decision, that the choice is ultimately yours, and you care about their input and help. This conversation demonstrates the maturity and responsibility most parents hope their teen embodies.

If you cannot talk to your parents about sex and proper protection/safety, never hesitate to take advantage of the abundance of resources available to you, such as Planned Parenthood, your doctor, or even a school nurse. Only take material regarding sex and safety from the Internet if it is from a credible/verifiable source to ensure you are being given accurate information.[a]

are safer to turn to, or simply know more and can give you better answers. Think about what is best for you in a particular situation and turn to the best people you can think of to get support.

Question:

How do I tell my mother I was molested? I don't want to lose her trust and I don't want to see her cry! Will she be mad at me?

—Sixteen-year-old

Answer:

Almost always mothers want their daughters to come and tell them when they have been hurt in some way. If you ask your mother for some private time with you and tell her you need to talk something over she will most likely sense that you are serious and she will do it. If you truly think that she would respond poorly you could tell someone else, a relative, a school counselor, a doctor, or a minister, and have them be with you when you tell your mother.

Sometimes moms are very concerned and upset and rather than being able to listen and show they care they become tearful or angry. They may want to get back at the person who did it or because they are worried they might say something like "How could you let that happen?" Usually this initial shock passes and moms can be a great help. Tell your mom what YOU need: to be held, to be listened to, or whatever. Keeping your troubles all to yourself is the worst thing because even if you try to forget about it, it is likely to continue bothering you.

Hang in there and good luck,

Health Professional, We Are Talking, teen health website[1]

Body Image

Sex and your body are very connected. After all, most times (unless you are engaging in phone sex or sending sexy messages or something like that) your body plays a huge role in a sexual encounter. So, it makes sense that thinking about sex will often make you think about your body.

The sad thing is a lot of people—especially young people—do not like their bodies. Eating disorders, fasting, and steroid use are all examples of how young people harm their bodies in order to change the way they look. In fact, over half of young women and almost a third of young men use unhealthy ways to control their weight, such as skipping meals, vomiting, and fasting.[2] Some young people will also start smoking, another unhealthy behavior, in order to try to lose weight. Why are so many people unhappy with the way they look?

For one thing, there is a myth that only beautiful people have sex or are worthy of sex; that only physically attractive people are sexual people or considered sexually desirable. This is simply not true. Humans are sexual beings. That means every person can be a sexual being. But, think about the images you see in the media in terms of who is considered sexy and who is involved in movie sex scenes: for the most part, those actors are skinny, cut, and smooth. They are small in all the right places and larger in all the right places. If we try to compare ourselves to the actors and models who are considered sex symbols, it's not easy to think of ourselves as good-looking or attractive. Then we might also think that we are not worthy of having a sexual or romantic relationship with another person. So, what can happen is that people try to change their bodies—through starving, taking steroids, or overexercising—in the hopes that they will become more attractive and therefore be more likely to have a sexual partner.

While it's true that most people like others who take care of themselves (you know, people who bathe, comb their hair, wash their face, wear clean and neat clothes, etc.), there is a huge variety of tastes when it comes to attractiveness. There are people who like super skinny folks, and there are those who prefer a person who is rounder, bulkier, or has more curves. Some people go gaga over strong arms, while others see a well-manicured hand as the biggest turn-on. The bottom line is, no matter how much you change your body to make it fit an ideal, there will be people out there who do not think you are attractive. And, no mat-

Songs That Celebrate Beauty

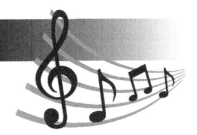

Here's a list of great songs that let us all know that beauty comes in all shapes and styles!

- "Fat Bottomed Girls" by Queen (1978)
- "Baby Got Back" by Sir Mix-a-Lot (1992)
- "Beautiful" by Christina Aguilera (2002)
- "Born This Way" by Lady Gaga (2013)
- "Perfect" by BJ The Chicago Kid (2014)
- "All about That Bass" by Meghan Trainor (2014)

ter what your body looks like, as long as you take care of what you have, there are people out there who will find you appealing. So, it's probably a better idea to focus on your natural look and on being a healthy and happy person instead of a media-defined "sexy one."

There is another connection between sex and body image that's pretty great. The more you are comfortable with your body, the more pleasurable and healthy your sexual experiences will be. If you are overly concerned about whether your partner thinks you look good, or if you wince if your partner grabs you by your "extra-chunky" middle to give you a kiss, it's hard to enjoy the time you are spending together. Instead of thinking about how your body looks while being sexual with a partner, pay attention to how it feels. Relax, enjoy the moment. Another way to feel more comfortable with your body is to explore it more. Masturbate or just touch yourself in different ways so you can figure out what does and doesn't feel good. Getting in touch with your sexual self when you're by yourself can help you discover what does and doesn't feel good to you. Nobody and no body is perfect—but the complete package sure as heck can be to that special someone.

Mental Health and Relationships

Having a mental health challenge can impact a sexual or romantic relationship in many ways. First, the condition itself may bring with it different characteristics such as feelings of stress, doubt, depression, or anxiety (among many other feelings) that can make it difficult to feel close to another. Also, some medications have "sexual side effects," which means the person taking them can experience decreased desires or abilities to have sex. There can be stigma attached to having a mental health challenge, and this may make it difficult for you or your partner to talk about how mental health plays a role in your relationship.

Deciding whether to disclose your mental health status to a romantic or sexual partner is a big decision. The fear of rejection can be huge. You need to be able to trust that person to understand what your mental health status means and how it might impact the relationship. If you are ready to disclose, it's a good idea to do it in a calm setting where you feel safe. Allow your partner to ask questions, but it's also important that your partner is listening to you and asking questions out of care and concern. Not all mental health challenges influence relationships, but they can and it's important to keep the communication open and free. A person who is in a relationship with someone with mental health challenges can be a good support. The couple might be able to go to appointments together; a partner not affected by mental health challenges may even talk to a provider to learn how to be a good support during difficult times.

Hopefully the two of you together will feel safe enough to ask and answer questions in order to best understand each other. A romantic partner can help a person feel calm and appreciate when a partner's mental health is affecting mood or ability to do things on a regular basis. At the same time, the person whose mental health is affecting the relationship also has a responsibility to communicate when things are difficult and not take negative emotions out on a partner.

Being in a relationship with someone with mental health challenges is not always easy. Having mental health challenges and being in a romantic relationship also has its difficulties. However, it is possible to have a fulfilling relationship if there is good communication, support, and understanding.

Dating Someone Older

While people of all genders can date someone older, most of the time when we think about an age difference between two people, we think about an older guy dating a younger female. However, age differences in all couples is something worth thinking about. If you are a young woman, you might already know the drill (others have probably heard this story, but might have less direct experience)—you meet a guy and the two of you really start to hit it off. The two of you seem to have so much in common, and your friends think he's great. You want to tell your mother about him, but you do not dare for one simple reason: he is older than you. You think your mother or father would freak if they knew how old he really is. You can hear their voices: "Older guys are only after one thing . . ." Well, how right are your folks? According to the research, girls with

Youth Speak Out: Dealing with Mental Health Issues in a Relationship, by Goose, Age 20

I am very honest about my mental health status with my romantic partner espe-cially since my mental health status has an impact on the relationship. When it comes to disclosing this information I usually evaluate when the right time to do it would be and I don't throw it all on the table at once because I don't want to overwhelm my partner. I allow my partner to ask any questions they have, and answer them as honestly as I can. Of course there are some things that I may not be ready to talk about but when I am ready I will.

My current partner has been there for me as much as she can. She has been understanding and patient with me. Sometimes she gets really worried and I have to reassure her that things are okay but I know that she does this out of love. She also knows that she can't just "fix" me. I think that for the most part we have learned enough about each other to be used to what one another needs and it has just become a part of our relationship. There are times where one of us is going through a rough time and the amount of support needed changes. One thing we had to learn was that sometimes the things we did had more to do with our mental health than the other person (decreased desire for sex, hard time communicating, easily upset, not wanting to be alone/wanting to be alone more). It's important for her to be able to know that my depression isn't a result of her not being able to make me happy.[b]

older boyfriends are more likely to experience pressure to have sex, are more likely to be forced to have sex when they didn't want to, and are more likely to have sex under the influence of alcohol and/or drugs.[3] In general, young people with older partners are less likely to practice safer sex and are more likely to become young parents.[4]

Not great things to hear. And these studies lead us to ask a logical question: If dating older guys seems like a bad idea according to both parents and the research, why does it happen so often? There are many possible reasons. First, females of-ten mature faster than males both physically and emotionally, so when a girl dates an older guy, she may be dating someone who has a similar level of maturity, or whose body has reached a similar developmental stage. But that reason would only account for a two, maybe three-year age difference.

Generally, no matter the gender of the two people, dating someone older can seem to have certain benefits. There can be a certain status associated with dating an older person. That person may have a job and thus be able to buy more things for you or in general. An older partner might have a car, which allows the couple more independence. An older partner may even have an apartment, which means it's easier for the couple to be alone together.

There could be some disadvantages to being with someone older. Older people might have more power over partners and may use this power to get what they want. By buying a younger partner things or providing a place to stay, the older partner may expect sexual favors in return (news flash: no one should expect sex in return for anything). An older partner may make the younger person feel that the older person is more sexually experienced and therefore gets to call the shots on where and when to have sex, and whether to practice safer sex. None of that is true—it's up to a couple to make sexual decisions together, and safer sex practices should always be used, no matter what. The bottom line is, status and power are not cool if they are held over people. If someone wants to control you, that is not a good relationship to be in.

If you are dating someone older, think about why you are dating this person. Then, think about why that person is dating you. Take time out to think about why a twenty-two-year-old would want to date a fifteen- or even seventeen-year-old. If the reasons seem shaky to you, that's because they are shaky. If control and power are a large part of the picture, it may be time to reconsider the relationship. Ask your friends—the ones you really trust—what they think. They'll tell you if the way your partner and you act doesn't seem fair or equal. Rely on your gut, too. Think deep down as to whether the relationship you are in is healthy. If you feel deep down that something is wrong with the relationship you are in, then something is wrong with that relationship. You have to feel comfortable dating who you are dating. If you are not, then the relationship is not right. Also, if you have to lie about your age to be in a relationship, that is not a good start to the partnership. Without honesty, a relationship will not go very far. The truth is bound to come out! Be true to yourself first, and if the relationship is right, it will hold strong. Then again, it's OK to start dating someone and then realize that person is not right for you.

Dating Someone Different

We all fall for a special someone for different reasons. While some people end up being with someone who shares a lot of similarities, others find themselves loving someone who is different from them when it comes to race, ethnicity, religion, or some other major characteristic. There are many benefits to partnering with

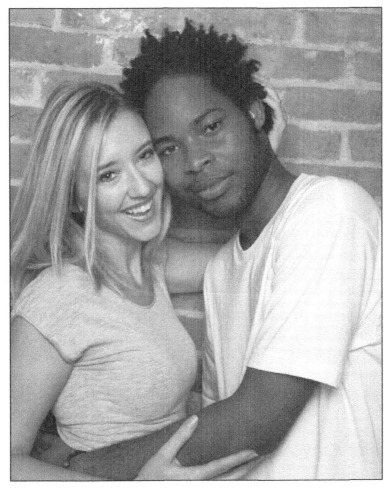

Dating someone different can make you grow as a person.

someone who is different. You may learn about a new culture or traditions that are different from your own. You might expand your ways of seeing and understanding the world by being exposed to different beliefs. By being close with someone from a different background than you are, you open yourself up to new experiences and, likewise, are able to share your culture and traditions with your partner, who can learn about you and your history. And, for the most part, young people are pretty accepting when two people who are different from each other partner up. For example, one survey found that more than half of high school students said they had dated someone of another race, while another 30 percent hadn't, but would consider it if the right person came along.[5]

On the other hand, there are challenges to dating someone who is of a different race, ethnicity, or religion. The two of you may disagree over some important things because of different value systems. Or you may find it difficult to understand each other because you were raised very differently and therefore see the world from diverse perspectives. While sometimes sincere conversations can help overcome those differences and compromises can be reached, sometimes fundamental differences will be too big for the relationship to last. It helps to really listen to each other to try to understand the other's point of view. Sometimes reading about your partner's culture can help, too. Ask for suggestions on how to educate yourself better when it comes to your partner's background, and offer similar resources in return.

Other challenges come from outside the relationship. There are people who will believe you are dating someone different from you because you have a fetish, not because your feelings for that person are sincere. Some people are flat-out afraid or prejudiced against people of certain backgrounds, and one or both of you may face that discrimination when you are together. People may look at you funny or disapprovingly as you walk down the street together. You might even hear direct comments from people who think you should "stick to your own kind."

Discrimination is all too real in our society. While it's true you and your partner can support each other, sometimes there are people in your community, school, or family who will not be supportive of your relationship. Open communication with your partner about your differences and how society perceives them will help both of you understand how to best be each other's ally.

Dealing with Family Members Who Can't Deal

If you are in a relationship with someone and family members don't approve of that person just because your partner is "different," here are some things you can do that might help your situation:

1. Ask those people why they do not feel that being close to someone of a particular race/ethnicity/religion is OK. Do not ask them about your relationship in particular—instead, focus on the general. Ask this question in a serious tone and with respect so that you can understand their position.
2. Explain your views on the issue. After you hear their side, calmly explain yours. Again, try not to get personal, but instead stay on a more general plane. Let them know that you have given a lot of thought to this issue and have your educated opinions. Even more impressive is to have some links to news stories or other articles written by experts to show that the reasons to fear an entire group of people are unfounded.
3. Talk about your friends of diverse backgrounds with your family. This shows your family members that you associate with people of different races, beliefs, and backgrounds in all parts of your life.

Television Couples That Model Differences

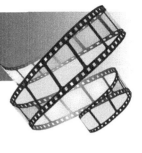

More than ever before, television series feature couples where the partners are different from each other. Here are just a few:

- Crosby and Jasmine on *Parenthood* (2010–2015) are an interracial couple. On *Empire* (2015–present), there's Andre and Rhonda. There are also interracial couples on *Scandal* (2012–present), *The Mindy Project* (2012–present), *New Girl* (2011–present)—the list goes on!
- On *NCIS* (2003–present), Tim McGee is living with his girlfriend, Delilah, who is in a wheelchair.
- *Broad City* (2014–present) features Ilana and Lincoln, who are from different religions.

4. Maybe have your family meet your partner, if you think it's safe and comfortable to do so—you certainly don't want to put your partner in a bad situation. Talk to your partner and to your family about the idea, separately. If your family seems to open up to the idea of you dating someone who has a different background from you, or at least is open to the idea that not everyone you associate with has to be like you, have your partner over for dinner (only if your partner likes the idea, too, of course). Make your parents see the wonderful person you have chosen to be with. The two of you together can demonstrate the respect and care you have for each other in a mature and responsible way.

Abortion

There are all sorts of opinions about abortion. Abortion is murder. Abortion is a woman's right to choose. Abortion is a sin. Abortion is safer than giving birth to a child. Depending on your point of view, all of these statements can be true. But, no matter who you are, having an abortion is not easy. Ending a pregnancy in this way will be emotionally difficult. You will remember this event for the rest of your life.

This doesn't mean that having an abortion is the wrong decision for you. It may be the right one; in your eyes it may be the only one. About one in four pregnancies in young people between the ages of fifteen and nineteen end in abortion.[6] Legally, only the person who is pregnant has a right to choose an abortion. The other half of the relationship has no legal right in the decision-making process. It would be nice if the two people who created the pregnancy could sit down to-

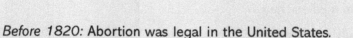

History of Abortion

Abortion laws have changed constantly throughout American history. Here is a very brief timeline of the major events that have influenced this issue.

- *Before 1820:* Abortion was legal in the United States.
- *1820:* Abortions after four months of pregnancy became illegal.
- *By 1900:* Most abortions were outlawed.
- *1965:* All abortions were outlawed.
- *1973:* The Supreme Court, under the *Roe v. Wade* decision, declared abortion legal because of our constitutional right to privacy.
- *1976:* The Supreme Court, under the *Planned Parenthood of Central Missouri v. Danforth*, declared it unconstitutional to demand a husband's permission if his wife wanted an abortion.
- *1977:* Through a series of decisions, the Supreme Court declared that public (in other words, government) funds did not have to be used to help pay for abortions.
- *1992:* The Supreme Court decided, in *Planned Parenthood of Southern Pennsylvania v. Casey*, that a state could require antiabortion materials to be distributed in clinics before a woman had an abortion and that a woman would have to return to the clinic twenty-four hours later in order to actually have the abortion.
- *2007:* In *Gonzalez v. Carhart*, the Supreme Court upheld a ban on "partial birth abortions" (this is not a medical term, but one used by the courts).[c]

gether and talk about options, but there's nothing in the law that states that this must happen. The person who is pregnant is the one who makes the decision.

A person under eighteen may not be able to legally make a decision about abortion without an adult's knowledge or consent. The laws about abortion vary from state to state as to whether or not a young person seeking an abortion needs to get permission from her parents (or a guardian, or relative) to have an abortion. They also vary on the level of permission needed, ranging from needing no permission or notification (in other words, parents do not even need to know that their child is getting an abortion), to needing full consent from *both* parents for the abortion, even if the parents are not together. As of 2016, thirty-eight states require some form of parental involvement when it comes to someone under eighteen getting an abortion.[7] You can find out about the laws in your state by calling a health clinic in your area or looking it up online.

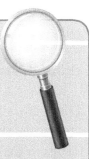

Think about It: Why It Might Be a Good Idea to Talk to Your Parents or Another Adult about Getting an Abortion

You may not want to tell a parent or other adult about an unintended pregnancy, but here are some reasons why it may be best to talk about it in the long run:

- Having an abortion is an intense experience. Hiding it from the trusted adults in your life could be very difficult.
- You could use an adult's support. Sure, the person you tell might be upset at first, but in the end the adults in your life may be able to help you through a tough time.
- Abortions are expensive—several hundred dollars—and insurance plans may or may not cover them. Talking to a trusted adult may get you the financial help you need.
- You might need a ride, help making an appointment, or the name of a trusted doctor.
- You could use a shoulder to cry on.

Some of you out there think that your parents would throw you out of the house or physically hurt you if you were to tell them that you were pregnant and thinking about getting an abortion. I'm not talking about those of you who think to yourself, "Oh my God, if my mom found out, she would kill me," upon receiving a bad grade on a report card or breaking a family heirloom while dusting. I'm referring to those of you out there who honestly would fear for your safety if your parents found out you were pregnant, never mind considering an abortion. For you, there is a way to get an abortion without getting guardian permission, no matter what state you live in, no matter what the law says. Through a process called judicial bypass, a young person can go to court and get the state's permission for an abortion. This is not an easy process, but for some it's the only option. A health clinic will help you understand the law better if you decide that this is something you need to look into. It's important to pursue this idea sooner rather than later though, as the process does take time and, when it comes to ending a pregnancy, time is a very important factor.

What Happens during an Abortion?

There are a few different types of abortion that can be broken down into two categories: surgical and medical. In this book, I only talk about the two simplest forms, as these are the most likely types you may encounter. The further the pregnancy progresses, the riskier the abortion procedure becomes. Although I am not suggesting that you should hurry your decision to have an abortion, having one more than four months into a pregnancy limits a person's options. At that point, the baby is more developed, and both the laws and the procedures become more complex.

Surgical Abortions

For pregnancies in the first trimester (up to twelve weeks), a procedure called suction-aspiration is performed. The patient lies down, with feet in stirrups like in a gynecological exam. Then, the cervix is numbed and stretched using smooth metal rods. Finally, a suction machine is inserted into the uterus, which pulls the fetus and placenta out. Although the procedure takes less than fifteen minutes, the whole appointment may last two to five hours because of the paperwork, questions, laboratory tests (to make sure a person really is pregnant), medications, anesthesia, procedure, recovery, and aftercare that's needed.

For pregnancies that are slightly further along (twelve to twenty-four weeks), the dilation and evacuation (D&E) procedure is performed. Although the actual procedure takes about thirty minutes, the person getting the abortion has to go to the clinic the day before to prepare for the procedure, so really the entire process takes two days. During the preparation on the first day, the doctor will dilate (enlarge) the cervix (opening of the uterus), by inserting a small rod or series of rods into the cervix. Overnight these rods gently expand, opening the entrance to the uterus. The next day, the patient goes back to the clinic for the abortion. During the abortion, the patient is put under general anesthesia, which means being "put under" while this is happening. The doctor uses a suction device to remove the fetus and may also use a curettage (an instrument used for scraping) to help remove the fetus. The patient will remain at the clinic for one to several hours to make sure everything is okay. If there is no heavy bleeding or other complications, it will be OK to leave. Some people, however, are kept overnight.

Medical Abortions

Medical abortions use various drugs to end a pregnancy, rather than relying on a medical procedure. Nevertheless, a person still needs to see a doctor in order to get a medical abortion. Some people refer to a medical abortion as taking "the abortion pill," but the reality is that taking a pill is only part of the process. A person who undergoes a medical abortion will first go to a doctor and take a pill, and then two days later go to the doctor again to get a vaginal suppository to complete the abortion process. Feeling nauseous and experiencing cramping are normal, but the doctor will tell you about possible side effects that signal any danger. After this second step, most pregnancies will end four to twenty-four hours later. Bleeding or spotting, however, can continue for up to two weeks more. Finally,

Helpful Hint

If you are considering counseling to get advice about whether to get an abortion, check that the counseling you seek is not antiabortion—people with an agenda can scare you into making a decision that you will later regret. Find someone with an open mind, someone who can help you consider *all* your legal options. Similarly, when you look for information online, try to use medical sites such as WebMD or the Mayo Clinic, which will provide you with factual information and statistics on abortions. If you do a general search, it's hard to differentiate fact from fiction.

the patient needs to see the doctor two weeks later to make sure that the abortion is complete, and there are no serious complications. This procedure is 92 to 95 percent effective and can be used during the first nine weeks of pregnancy.

Going through a medical abortion is the same as getting a surgical abortion, from a legal standpoint. That means, all the laws about minors getting abortions in your state will apply to medical abortions, too. For more information on this and other abortion issues, visit www.naral.org.

Adoption

Sometimes women who are pregnant but not ready to be parents do not believe in abortion, do not want an abortion, or cannot have an abortion. For these people, placing the baby for adoption is a possible solution to pregnancy. Overall, it is very uncommon for young people to decide to give their babies for adoption—only about 5 percent of pregnant teens choose this option.[8] It's not easy to decide to place a baby for adoption, and it's important to remember that adoption is permanent. Because adoption is such an important decision, think about why you're considering this option. If the reasons you list are temporary, then you might want to consider living through some tough times in order to keep this little person-to-be in your life.

If the situations you are facing are more permanent, or you are absolutely certain that you cannot take care of a child any time soon, then considering adoption might be a good idea. But before you make your decision, make sure that you do not do it alone. Both halves of the couple who created the pregnancy ideally will talk about their options together. Talking to family members, a counselor, a religious leader, or other trusted adult can help you see what support you may or may not have if you decide to keep the baby. A young person cannot take care of a child alone; it takes friends, loved ones, and money. If you don't have these resources, taking care of a child is close to impossible.

If you decide that you want to place a baby for adoption, look up adoption services online that are in your area or in the nearest city. You'll see many choices—some are for-profit, some not-for-profit, and some even focus on specific religions and ethnicities. If it's important to you that the child has parents of the same racial and/or religious background as you, ask the adoption agency if it has parents of your background on the waiting list. Choose the adoption agency that you think is right for you, or call a few to see which you think is best (see the list of questions to ask about the adoption agency and the potential family of the baby).

There are two types of adoption: closed (or confidential) and open. In a closed adoption, the birth parents and the adoptive parents never know each other. The

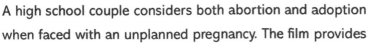

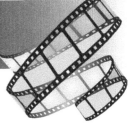

Movie Review: Juno (2007, 1h 36m)

A high school couple considers both abortion and adoption when faced with an unplanned pregnancy. The film provides a great look into how complicated, but rewarding, the adoption process can be.

only information the adoptive parents have about their new baby is important medical information so that they can make sure their baby gets the best care possible. In open adoptions, the two sets of parents know something about each other. What and how much they know about each other can vary a lot. At a minimum, the birth mother can pick the adoptive parent(s) by reading some profiles and choosing the best family. At the most, the birth mother will stay in contact with the adoptive parent(s) as the child grows up. She can write, call, and even visit the baby and new family. Not all states allow open adoptions; go online or call an adoption agency near you to see what types of open adoptions are available in your state. If you are under eighteen, the laws might be different so make sure you get all the facts and know your rights. As of 2016, forty states allow a minor to place a child for adoption, but some require a legal adult to be involved in some capacity.[9] Check out adoption.com to learn more.

Questions to Consider

Once you decide to place the baby you are carrying for adoption, you'll still have many questions to ask and answer yourself. Every time you meet with someone regarding the adoption, make a list of questions beforehand, as the meetings can be intense and stressful; there might be a lot of emotions involved. Here are some questions that will help you get started. Feel free to add some of your own.

Questions to ask the adoption agency about the adoptive family:

- Why do the people want to adopt a baby right now? Are there other children in the adoptive family's home?
- What kind of life do they lead right now? What kind of recreation or hobbies do they enjoy?
- What are the adoptive family's values? Do they have strong religious beliefs?

- How will the adoptive family take care of the baby? Will the baby be in day care or will someone stay home with the child?
- What is the adoptive family's view on disciplining a child?
- Is there a large extended family to help take care of the child?

Here are some questions to ask yourself:

- Do I care what religion the adoptive family follows?
- Do I care about the racial or ethnic backgrounds of the adoptive family?
- Do I want my child to have older brothers or sisters?
- Do I want the adoptive family to live near me?

Questions for potential parents (if you are in a position to ask them—or see if the adoption agency will ask them for you):

- Do you have any experience with children?
- What do your families think about your adopting a baby?
- Will you tell the child about the adoption? When and how?
- What will you tell the child about me?
- What are your religious beliefs?
- What are your beliefs about education?
- What forms of discipline will you use with the child?
- Are you willing to maintain contact with me as your child grows up?
- What type of contact are you most comfortable with? How often would you like to stay in contact with me?
- Can I send the child cards, messages, or small gifts on birthdays and holidays?[10]

Alternative Sexual Behaviors

Alternative sexual behaviors are things people do to turn themselves on that are not considered traditional sexual activities such as kissing, touching, and oral, anal, and vaginal sex. These more commonly known sexual activities in and of themselves are often forbidden topics to discuss—when you have questions about a certain sexual practice that is labeled "alternative," it becomes next to impossible to find reliable information about it. Thinking and learning about alternative sexual behaviors does not make you abnormal or a freak. Discovering that you like some of them does not mean anything is wrong with you. As with other sexual activities, alternative sexual behaviors done in a safe, consensual, mature, and responsible manner do not have to have such negative or strange reputations. Read on to learn more.

Fetishes

The term *fetish* is often misunderstood and used improperly. A fetish, in medical and psychological terms, is an object that someone *needs* in order to get sexually aroused. The object actually takes the place of a human in terms of sexual feelings and interactions (that is, a person would rather be sexual *with* the shoe than the person wearing it). A person who has a true fetish is not able to have a sexual relationship with another human being. A person who has a true fetish should talk to a counselor or doctor about getting help so that healthy relationships can be established with people, not things.

What most people think of when they think of fetishes are really "turn-ons." There are as many turn-ons out there as there are people. Some of the more common ones are certain types of clothing, such as high heels; different materials, such as leather or spandex; a certain color hair or a certain occupation (nurse, police officer, etc.). For the most part, these sexual turn-ons and preferences are a private matter that you may choose to share with a serious sexual partner. Or you may decide to keep them completely to yourself and have them stay in a fantasy. Be careful about sharing fetishes with any random person—they could be used against you for humor. Many people find anything even remotely sexual funny. If disrespectful people find out that you are sexually aroused by anything that does not fit under their own definition of sexy, it can become a reason to make fun of you (and we all know that making fun of other people really isn't acceptable as a general rule). In truth, one person's turn-on is another person's turnoff, and there is nothing inherently wrong with that. Exploring what you do and do not like sexually is a healthy way to get to know yourself better. Over time, and with the right person, you may want to share your turn-ons with special others who are worthy of knowing about that part of you.

Shaving

Looking at images of naked people online and in pornographic magazines, for example, one could easily think that all people shave their genitals and many other parts of their bodies. This is simply not true; many people choose to keep their pubic hair either trimmed neatly or let it go completely natural. There are many benefits to keeping pubic hair. Pubic hair provides a protective barrier between you and your clothing (less chafing!), keeps your genital region cleaner and freer of bacteria, and decreases the chances of yeast infections and skin breakdown. Humans have pubic hair for many good reasons! If you do, however, decide to shave your pubic hair, you should do it for you—not because someone says you should. After all, it's your hair that's going to itch like crazy when it grows back.

Multiple Partners/Sharing/Threesomes

Having multiple partners at one time might sound appealing, but it's pretty darn complicated. Therefore, my advice to you is do not engage in a threesome. These sorts of relationships and sexual experiences can only end in a big mess of drama, confusion, hurt feelings, and destroyed relationships. Sure, they may seem like fun in your fantasy world, but that is where they should stay—in the fantasy world. In pornography, group sex and orgies look fun and sensual, but those situations are carefully choreographed and rehearsed, so that when you watch them, no one is feeling left out of the action or concerned about what is happening when the focus is on someone else. Also, the people in these movies do not have to hang out with each other the next day. They just collect their paychecks and carry on with their lives. No mess, no confusion, no reality. There are some older adults who are able to love more than one person and maintain healthy relationships with small groups or a couple of individuals. This sort of arrangement, however, requires a lot of communication and openness when it comes to sharing feelings, boundaries, and rules regarding safer sex practices.

Power Relationships

There are all sorts of relationships and relationship activities that fall under this category. Platonically, a parent–child relationship has power issues that go along with it, as does a boss–employee relationship. What a "power relationship" means in a college human sexuality textbook is a sexual or romantic relationship that has an unequal power status *through the consent of both people involved.* That is a very important part of a mature power relationship; it is agreed to by both parts of the couple. In fact, the relationship is so consensual, that the two people will sit down and write a contract together so that they have a very solid understanding about what the relationship is and isn't, and what is and is not OK when it comes to what happens in the relationship. Safety is the top priority in a mature power relationship.

Fantasy and role play (when people pretend to be people they are not, or pretend to be in a place they are not) is often, but not always, involved. A lot of people will talk about BDSM, or B&D and S&M. In these abbreviations, B = bondage, D = discipline, S = sadism, and M = masochism. Bondage is when people are restrained with ropes or something else during sexual activity. Discipline is when strict rules are set in a sexual relationship, and "punishment," which is agreed upon in the contract described earlier, is administered when these rules are violated. This punishment is seen as pleasurable to both the giver and the recipient. Sadism is feeling sexual pleasure in hurting someone in a way that

that person has agreed to in a contract, and masochism is feeling sexual pleasure when one receives that pain—again, in a way that was previously agreed to in a written contract.

The idea of power relationships has become more visible in popular culture since the very popular book and movie *50 Shades of Grey* came out. In this story, a young woman enters into a power relationship with an older man by signing a contract. However, that's where the similarities to BDSM stop. There is nothing healthy in a relationship where one person stalks the other—tracking the other down at work or when the partner is out with her parents, or following the partner uninvited to another state. There is nothing healthy when someone says yes to sex that person is uncomfortable with. *50 Shades of Grey* is about manipulation and an abuse of power, not about a loving relationship. As with threesomes or group sex, I again urge you not to engage in any type of sexual power relationship—and certainly don't use *50 Shades of Grey* as an example of how to be in a relationship with someone else. The logistics of a true power relationship are very complex, and the activities can be very dangerous if done by people who do not know exactly what they are doing. While fantasizing about different types of power in a relationship is fine, it's best to keep those ideas in your mind and not try to actually do them with another person.

Alcohol, Drugs, and Sex

Combining alcohol or drugs with sexual activity is challenging to think about. There are some people who feel that they need to be "on something"—alcohol or another drug—in order to open up sexually. These people believe that alcohol lowers their inhibitions and gets them to relax, which might allow them to feel more comfortable talking about, engaging in, or initiating sexual activities. However, the effects of drinking and drugs on sexual performance and sexual safety are enormous. For this reason, I believe it is best not to combine alcohol and drugs with any sexual activity.

The main reason it's not a good idea to combine sex and alcohol and other drugs is because when people are under the influence of something, they may not be able to give consent or understand clearly whether someone is consenting. Without clear and enthusiastic consent, no sexual activity should take place. Therefore, the very simple approach to healthy sexuality is to not mix sex and alcohol or any other substance, because doing so can substantially increase the chances of having sex without consent, which by definition is sexual assault.

There are other reasons not to combine sex with substance use. Consider the following:

- People of any age, but especially younger people, are less likely to use condoms (or use them properly if they do use them) while under the influence. Not using a condom increases the chances of getting a sexually transmitted disease or having an unplanned pregnancy. In fact, one study found that almost half of all unplanned teen pregnancies happened as a result of sex under the influence of alcohol or drugs.[11]
- People who are under the influence of drugs or alcohol lose their ability to consent to sex. Having sex with someone without consent is rape.
- In the short term, being under the influence can make it impossible to have an erection or have the body be biologically ready for sex.

If having sex under the influence of either alcohol or drugs is so bad for you, why do so many people do it? There is a lot of pressure out there to have sex. Some of this pressure comes from the media, some comes from your friends, and some of it comes from inside of you. There is a part of you that wants to have sex, but another part of you that doesn't want to have sex. The reasons that you want to have sex might be curiosity, desire, you're in love, to get props, it feels good, or because it sounds like fun. The reasons you have for believing you should not have sex can range from "I do not believe sex before marriage is right," to "I just don't know this person well enough," to "It would be fun, but I already have a partner." Other reasons to not want to have sex are "I'm just not feeling it," "I don't feel ready," or "I feel like I'm being pressured." So, you have this debate going on in your head about whether to have sex; what better way to end the debate than to eliminate one of the sides? By drinking or using drugs, the side that says you shouldn't have sex sometimes disappears. End of debate, but possibly the beginning of a lot of problems.

Some of the reasons that some people have sex while under the influence depend on their gender. For young women, alcohol can be seen as an excuse to express their sexuality and sexual desires. This is because there is a myth that girls and women who are sexually active, or who express sexual desire, are sluts (see chapter 10 for more thoughts on this). Therefore, a young woman may not want to simply say to another person, or even to herself, that she is feeling sexual. But, that same young woman may think that if she gets drunk, it's OK to express her sexuality. Her flirting, desires, and other sexual behaviors can now be blamed on the alcohol instead of her personality: this person is not really a slut; she is just drunk, or high, or whatever. However, someone who is expressing her sexuality is not doing anything wrong or shameful—it's natural to have sexual desires, no matter who you are. Also, just because someone is flirting or acting sexual does not mean sex is desired. A person always has to consent to sexual activity.

For young men, alcohol can be a crutch to help them through a sexual encounter. There's a myth out there that guys are supposed to want sex all the time, even though that's not true—no one wants sex all the time. But what happens when a guy knows that he should not have sex or doesn't want to have sex, for whatever reason? This guy should choose not to have sex, but that does not always happen. This is because the guy also knows that a young man who does not want sex or turns down a sexual proposition might be seen as a loser in the eyes of society and possibly his peers (again, chapter 10 has more about this). Being under the influence of alcohol or another drug might make a guy believe that he wants to have the sex he is "supposed" to have. Losing sobriety might silence his desires not to have sex that contradict the social messages that say he should be having sex. Also, a guy might believe that being a little tipsy might help him take potential rejection a bit more easily—this is another myth; rejection is hard, no matter what state you are in. Again, it's important to say that being sexual with someone under the influence—no matter how that person is acting—is wrong because it means you are being sexual with someone who has not given proper consent.

The bottom line is that sex and alcohol or drugs is a typical but potentially unhealthy combination. If you don't think you would be able to have sex without being under the influence of a substance, think again about having sex. If you are thinking of being sexual with someone who is under the influence of drugs or alcohol—don't. The best sex is always sex where both people are absolutely certain that both are completely into it.

Conclusion

When it comes to knowing all you need to know about sex and relationships, this book barely covers the basics. There's so much to know, and every person has different needs for different information. However, I do hope this book helps you better understand that you have already experienced a lot in your life; I also hope it encourages you to keep learning about things that are important to you or just plain interesting. Asking questions about sex can only make you wiser.

Keep this book around as a reference, in case you forget some of the facts you read. Reread sections when the time is right to revisit certain concepts. I would love it if you recommended or passed this book along to a friend or family member if there's someone out there you care about who might find it interesting or useful.

My goals for writing this book were to help young people think about how they feel when it comes to different aspects of sexuality and relationships. I also want to encourage them to make responsible sexual decisions that reflect their feelings, values, and who they are. Ultimately, you're the one who will decide what you want to do and what you don't want to do sexually. You are the one who will set your sexual values. All this book can offer is facts, different perspectives, and suggestions to make your decisions more informed.

I leave you with some final words of advice as you continue your sexual journey:

- Whenever you are sexual with another person, make sure both of you are consenting to whatever it is that you're doing. It's important to get your partner's consent, and it's important that your partner gets yours.
- If you're forced to be sexual in any way against your will, you are not at fault. If this happens, I hope you find someone who will support you.
- Listen to your partner when you're in a relationship. Listening is a powerful way to get to know someone better and to grow together intimately.
- Listen to yourself. Trust your gut. If something doesn't feel right, comfortable, or good, take a step back. Give yourself time to think about what it is that is making you feel uneasy. Respect those feelings and don't let anyone pressure you into doing something that you know is wrong for you.

- You are an amazing person. No matter your gender, sexual orientation, sexual preferences—you are worthy of having a wonderful relationship with someone who respects you, loves you, and sees you as the beautiful person you are. Don't settle. Partners build each other up, and you deserve to be with someone who makes you feel fantastic.

Best of luck!

Notes

Introduction

1. This model of sexuality education was first developed in Europe and is explained more fully at Advocates for Youth at http://www.advocatesforyouth.org/the-3rs.

---

a. Advocates for Youth, "Comprehensive Sex Education: Research and Results," 2009, http://www.advocatesforyouth.org/storage/advfy/documents/fscse.pdf. Accessed May 5, 2016.
b. See Richard Burton (translator), *The Kama Sutra of Vatsyayana* (Mineola, NY: Dover, 2006; originally published 1883), www.sacred-texts.com/sex/kama/kama101.htm. Accessed May 5, 2016.

Chapter 1

1. M. Warren and A. C. Petersen, *Girls at Puberty*, ed. J. Brooks-Gunn and A. C. Petersen (New York: Plenum Press, 1983).
2. Unless otherwise noted, all questions and answers are provided by the We Are Talking teen health website. These questions and answers were submitted by young people via the site's web address, pamf.org/teen, and answered by doctors from the We Are Talking website.
3. N. H. Alzubaidi, H. L. Chapin, V. H. Vanderhoof, K. A. Calis, and L. M. Nelson, "Meeting the Needs of Young Women with Secondary Amenorrhea and Spontaneous Premature Ovarian Failure," *Obstetrics & Gynecology* 99 (2002): 720–725.
4. Demelza Needham, Martine Carroll, Emileen Ng, and Stine Braathen, "History of PMS in Western Society," *Premenstrual Syndrome*, 2001, remus.artsmmc.uwa.edu.au/www-projects/anth228328/meds/history.html. Accessed May 22, 2002.
5. S. A. Rathus, J. S. Nevid, and L. Fichner-Rathus, *Human Sexuality in a World of Diversity* (Boston, MA: Allyn and Bacon, 2002), 101–104.
6. The National Campaign to Prevent Teen and Unplanned Pregnancy, "Teen Pregnancy and High School Dropout: What Communities Can Do to Address These Issues," n.d., https://thenationalcampaign.org/sites/default/files/resource-primary-download/teen-preg-hs-dropout-summary.pdf. Accessed May 2, 2016.
7. Full citation: Jessica Akin, *Pregnancy and Parenting: The Ultimate Teen Guide*, It Happened to Me, no. 48 (Lanham, MD: Rowman & Littlefield, 2016).
8. UNAIDS, "Male Circumcision: Context, Criteria and Culture," February 26, 2007, http://www.unaids.org/en/resources/presscentre/featurestories/2007/february/20070226mcpt1 (Accessed online May 2, 2016).
9. UNAIDS, "Male Circumcision."
10. From L. K. Gowen's personal archives of online questions and her responses.

a. H. Finley, www.mum.org. Accessed July 7, 2002.

b. Guttmacher Institute, "American Teens' Sexual and Reproductive Health," May 2014, https://www.guttmacher.org/sites/default/files/factsheet/fb-atsrh.pdf. Accessed May 2, 2016.

Chapter 2

1. Sabra Katz-Wise, "Sexual Fluidity in Young Adult Women and Men: Associations with Sexual Orientation and Sexual Identity Development," *Psychology & Sexuality* 6 (2015): 189–208.
2. GLSEN, "The 2013 National School Climate Survey: Executive Summary," 2013, http://www.glsen.org/article/2013-national-school-climate-survey. Accessed October 6, 2016.
3. GLSEN, "The 2013 National School Climate Survey."

a. Essay written on March 24, 2016, by "Kellyn." Pseudonym chosen to protect anonymity.

Chapter 3

1. *Merriam-Webster Dictionary*, s.v. "abstain," http://www.merriam-webster.com/dictionary/abstain. Accessed October 6, 2016.
2. SIECUS, *Teens Talk about Sex: Adolescent Sexuality in the 90s* (New York: SIECUS, 1994), 24.

a. R. Brasch, *How Did Sex Begin? The Sense and Nonsense of Sexual Customs and Traditions* (Australia: Angus and Roberts, 1995), 16–19.
b. Reprinted with permission from the *Rational Enquirer*. Oregon Teen Pregnancy Task Force. Issues available online at https://public.health.oregon.gov/HealthyPeopleFamilies/Youth/Pages/re.aspx.

Chapter 4

1. Centers for Disease Control and Prevention, "YRBSS Results," 2013, http://www.cdc.gov/healthyyouth/data/yrbs/results.htm. Accessed May 2, 2016.
2. SIECUS, *Teens Talk about Sex: Adolescent Sexuality in the 90s* (New York: SIECUS, 1994), 18.
3. K. Conklin, *Adolescent Sexual Behavior: Demographics* (Washington, DC: Advocates for Youth, 2012), http://www.advocatesforyouth.org/publications/publications-a-z/413-adolescent-sexual-behavior-i-demographics. Accessed July 9, 2016.
4. Centers for Disease Control and Prevention, "Chlamydia—CDC Fact Sheet," last updated May 19, 2016, http://www.cdc.gov/std/chlamydia/stdfact-chlamydia.htm. Accessed October 6, 2016.
5. Sara A. Vasilenko, Megan K. Maas, and Eva S. Lefkowitz, "'It Felt Good but Weird at the Same Time:' Emerging Adults' First Experiences of Six Different Sexual Behaviors," *Journal of Adolescent Research* 30 (2015): 586–606.

6. Unless otherwise noted, all questions and answers are provided by the We Are Talking teen health website. These questions and answers were submitted by young people via the web address, pamf.org/teen, and answered by doctors from the We Are Talking website.
7. D. P. Welsh, C. M. Grello, and M. S. Harper, "No Strings Attached: The Nature of Casual Sex in College Students," *Journal of Sex Research* 43 (2006): 255–267.
8. C. M. Grello and D. P. Welsh, "The Nature of Adolescents' Non-Romantic Sexual Relationships and Their Link with Well-Being," poster presented at the ninth biennial meeting of the Society for Research on Adolescence, New Orleans, Louisiana, April 2002.

a. Essay and chart written by Sofie Ofelia. Sent to the author via email on January 23, 2016.
b. Visit Al Vernacchio's TED talk, "Sex Needs a New Metaphor. Here's One," at https://www.ted.com/talks/al_vernacchio_sex_needs_a_new_metaphor_here_s_one?language=en. Accessed May 20, 2016.
c. J. H. Kellogg, *Plain Facts for Old and Young: Embracing the Natural History and Hygiene of Organic Life.* Made available by the Internet Archive, https://archive.org/details/plainfaorold-00kell. Accessed May 2, 2016.
d. E. M. Duvall, *Facts of Life and Love for Teen-Agers* (Chicago: All Popular Library, 1957), 75.

Chapter 5

1. American Sexual Health Association, "Statistics," n.d., http://www.ashasexualhealth.org/stdsstis/statistics/. Accessed May 2, 2016.
2. Centers for Disease Control and Prevention, "STDs in Adolescents and Young Adults," last reviewed January 7, 2014, http://www.cdc.gov/std/stats12/adol.htm. Accessed May 2, 2016.
3. Unless otherwise noted, all questions and answers are provided by the We Are Talking teen health website. These questions and answers were submitted by young people via the web address, pamf.org/teen, and answered by doctors from the We Are Talking website.
4. Kaiser Family Foundation, *National Survey of Teens on HIV/AIDS* (Washington, DC: Henry J. Kaiser Family Foundation, 2000), https://kaiserfamilyfoundation.files.wordpress.com/2013/01/national-survey-of-teens-on-hiv-aids.pdf. Accessed May 2, 2016.

Chapter 6

1. WebMD, "I Forgot to Take My Birth Control Pill. Now What?" May 17, 2014, http://www.webmd.com/sex/birth-control/forgot-to-take-your-birth-control-pills. Accessed July 9, 2016.
2. Valerie French, "A Quick Guide to Skipping Periods with Birth Control," Bedsider, September 19, 2013, https://bedsider.org/features/290-a-quick-guide-to-skipping-periods-with-birth-control. Accessed July 9, 2016.

a. Jennifer S. Manlove, Suzanne Ryan, and Kerry Franzetta, "Contraceptive Use and Consistency in U.S. Teenagers' Most Recent Sexual Relationships," *Perspectives on Sexual and Reproductive Health* 36 (2004): 265–275.

b. Unless otherwise noted, all questions and answers are provided by the We Are Talking teen health website. These questions and answers were submitted by young people via the web address, pamf.org/teen, and answered by doctors from the We Are Talking website.

Chapter 7

1. R. A. Spitz, "Hospitalism: An Inquiry into the Genesis of Psychiatric Conditions in Early Childhood," *Psychoanalytic Study of the Child* 1 (1945): 53–74, and R. A. Spitz, "Hospitalism: A Follow-Up Report on Investigation Described in Volume I, 1945," *Psychoanalytic Study of the Child* 2 (1946): 113–117.

a. M. J. Zimmer-Gembeck, J. Siebenbrunner, and W. A. Collins, "Diverse Aspects of Dating: Associations with Psychosocial Functioning from Early to Middle Adolescence," *Journal of Adolescence* 24, no. 3 (June 2001): 313–336.
b. Reprinted with permission from the *Rational Enquirer* (2016) by the Oregon Teen Pregnancy Task Force.
c. From L. K. Gowen's personal archives of online questions and her responses.

Chapter 8

1. Emmeline May and Blue Seat Studios, "Consent: It's Simple as Tea," YouTube video, May 12, 2015, https://www.youtube.com/watch?v=oQbei5JGiT8. Accessed May 2, 2016. Warning: This video contains the F-bomb.

a. Associated Press, "California: Sexual Consent Lessons Now Required," *New York Times*, October 1, 2015, http://www.nytimes.com/2015/10/02/us/california-sexual-consent-lessons -now-required.html?_r=0. Accessed May 2, 2016.
b. Suzanne Ryan, Kerry Franzetta, Jennifer S. Manlove, and Emily Holcombe, "Adolescents' Discussions about Contraception or STDs with Partners before First Sex," *Perspectives on Sexual and Reproductive Health* 39 (2007): 149—157.
c. From L. K. Gowen's personal archives of online questions and her responses.

Chapter 9

1. Love Is Respect, "Dating Abuse Statistics," n.d., http://www.loveisrespect.org/resources/ dating-violence-statistics/. Accessed May 3, 2016.
2. David Finkelhor, Anne Shattuck, Heather A. Turner, and Sherry L. Hamby, "The Lifetime Prevalence of Child Sexual Abuse and Sexual Assault Assessed in Late Adolescence," *Journal of Adolescent Health* 30 (2014): 1–5, http://www.unh.edu/ccrc/pdf/9248.pdf. Accessed May 3, 2016.
3. Women Helping Women, "Teen Dating Violence," n.d., http://www.womenhelpingwomen .org/what-is-abuse/teen-dating-violence/. Accessed May 3, 2016.

4. RAINN, "The Offenders," n.d., https://rainn.org/get-information/statistics/sexual-assault -offenders. Accessed May 3, 2016.
5. RAINN, "Reporting Rates," n.d., https://rainn.org/get-information/statistics/reporting -rates. Accessed May 3, 2016.

Chapter 10

1. Kate H. Rademacher, *Media, Sex, and Health: A Community Guide for Professionals and Parents* (Chapel Hill, NC: Women's Center, 2007), http://compassctr.org/wp-content/uploads/2012/11/Mediamanual2007compressed.pdf. Accessed May 2, 2016.
2. Rademacher, *Media, Sex, and Health.*
3. Dale Kunkel, Keren Eyal, Keli Finnerty, Erica Biely, and Edward Donnerstein, *Sex on TV* (Santa Barbara, CA: Kaiser Family Foundation, 2004), 35.
4. Unless otherwise noted, all questions and answers are provided by the We Are Talking teen health website. These questions and answers were submitted by young people via the web address, pamf.org/teen, and answered by doctors from the We Are Talking website.

a. National Public Radio, "Is '16 And Pregnant' an Effective Form of Birth Control?" *All Things Considered*, last modified January 13, 2014, http://www.npr.org/2014/01/13/262175399/is -16-and-pregnant-an-effective-form-of-birth-control. Accessed May 2, 2016.

Chapter 11

1. Amanda Lenhart, *Teens and Sexting* (Washington, DC: Pew Research Center, 2009), http://www.pewinternet.org/files/old-media//Files/Reports/2009/PIP_Teens_and_Sexting.pdf. Accessed May 3, 2016.
2. Julia R. Lippman and Scott W. Campbell, "Damned If You Do, Damned If You Don't . . . If You're a Girl: Relational and Normative Contexts of Adolescent Sexting in the United States," *Journal of Children and Media* 8, no. 4, (2014): 371–386, DOI: 10.1080/17482798 .2014.923009.
3. Justin Patchin, "You Received a Sext, Now What? Advice for Teens," Cyberbullying Research Center, last updated February 2, 2011. http://cyberbullying.org/you-received-a-sext -now-what-advice-for-teens/. Accessed May 3, 2016.
4. K. H. Robinson, P. Bansel, N. Denson, G. Ovenden, and C. Davies, "Growing Up Queer: Issues Facing Young Australians Who Are Gender Variant and Sexuality Diverse," Young and Well Cooperative Research Centre, Melbourne, February 27, 2014, http://www.glhv. org.au/report/growing-queer-issues-facing-young-australians-who-are-gender-variant-and-sexuality-diverse. Accessed October 6, 2016.

a. Essay written by Olivia Yokas. Essay emailed to author on March 31, 2016.
b. Peter G. Polos, Sushanth Bhat, Divya Gupta, Richard J. O'Malley, Vincent A. DeBari, Hinesh Upadhyay, Saqib Chaudhry, Anitha Nimma, Genevieve Pinto-Zipp, and Sudhansu Chokrovertya, "The impact of Sleep Time-Related Information and Communication Technology

(STRICT) on Sleep Patterns and Daytime Functioning in American Adolescents," *Journal of Adolescence* 44 (2015): 234–244.

c. Cyber Civil Rights Initiative, www.cybercivilrights.org. Accessed May 3, 2016.

Chapter 12

1. Unless otherwise noted, all questions and answers are provided by the We Are Talking teen health website. These questions and answers were submitted by young people via its web address, pamf.org/teen, and answered by doctors from the We Are Talking website.
2. D. Neumark-Sztainer, *I'm, Like, SO Fat!* (New York: Guilford Press), 5.
3. L. Kris Gowen, S. Shirley Feldman, Rafael Diaz, and Donnovan Somera Yisrael, "Comparison of the Sexual Behaviors and Attitudes of Adolescent Girls with Older vs. Similar-Aged Boyfriends," *Journal of Youth and Adolescence* 33 (2004): 167–175.
4. Jennifer Manlove, Elizabeth Terry-Humen, and Erum Ikramullah, "Young Teenagers and Older Sexual Partners: Correlates and Consequences for Males and Females," *Perspectives on Sexual and Reproductive Health* 38 (2006): 197–207.
5. K. S. Peterson, "Interracial Dating Is No Big Deal for Teens," *USA Today*, November 3, 1997, A10.
6. Kathryn Kost and Stanley Henshaw, *U.S. Teenage Pregnancies, Births and Abortions, 2010: National and State Trends by Age, Race and Ethnicity* (New York: Guttmacher Institute, 2014), https://www.guttmacher.org/sites/default/files/report_pdf/ustptrends10.pdf. Accessed May 16, 2016.
7. Guttmacher Institute, "An Overview of Abortion Laws," last updated May 1, 2016, http://www.guttmacher.org/statecenter/spibs/spib_OAL.pdf. Accessed May 16, 2016.
8. SexInfo Online, "Teen Pregnancy Options," last updated January 31, 2012, http://www.soc.ucsb.edu/sexinfo/article/teen-pregnancy-options. Accessed May 16, 2016.
9. Guttmacher Institute, "State Policies in Brief: Minors' Rights as Parents," last updated March 1, 2016, http://www.guttmacher.org/statecenter/spibs/spib_MRP.pdf. Accessed May 16, 2016.
10. These questions were provided and used with permission by www.birthmother.com, during the first writing of this book.
11. Cited in S. Foster, "Early Use of Booze, Drugs Leads to Sex and Problems," *San Diego Union-Tribune*, January 23, 2000.

a. Reprinted with permission from the *Rational Enquirer* by the Oregon Teen Pregnancy Prevention Task Force. Issues available online at https://public.health.oregon.gov/HealthyPeople Families/Youth/Pages/re.aspx.
b. Essay written by "Goose" and sent to author via email on February 12, 2016. Name has been changed to protect anonymity.
c. American Civil Liberties Union, "Timeline of Important Reproductive Cases Decided by the Supreme Court," https://www.aclu.org/timeline-important-reproductive-freedom-cases -decided-supreme-court. Accessed May 16, 2016.

Resources

Need more information? Check out these books, websites, video channels, and hot lines to get the facts you may need when certain issues come up or you just want more information.

Books

Bell, R. *Changing Bodies, Changing Lives*. New York: Random House, 1998. The book is so big because it has it all. Yes, it is a little outdated, but there is still a lot of good information not only on sex and sexuality, but also substance use, eating disorders, and your emotions.

Corinna, H. *S.E.X.: The All-You-Need-to-Know Sexuality Guide to Get You through Your Teens and Twenties*. 2nd ed. Boston: Da Capo Lifelong Books, 2016. This book is written by the creator of the amazing Scarlet Teen website (listed later in these resources). It covers a lot about relationships as well as sexual health, and is very inclusive of all sexual and gender orientations.

Huegel, K. *GLBTQ: The Survival Guide for Gay, Lesbian, Bisexual, Transgender, and Questioning Teens*. Minneapolis: Free Spirit Publishing, 2011. This is a great book for anyone thinking about their sexual orientation or gender identity, or who simply wants to learn more about these topics. It covers everything from dating to homophobia to your rights in school. It also has a chapter on religion.

Lopez, R. I. *The Teen Health Book: A Parent's Guide to Adolescent Health and Well-Being*. New York: W. W. Norton, 2002. Sure, it is written for parents, but this book, written by a doctor, has a lot of good facts written in pretty clear language.

Orenstein, P. *Girls and Sex: Navigating the Complicated New Landscape*. New York: Harper, 2016. Journalist Peggy Orenstein has written some pretty great books about females and sexuality such as *School Girls*, and *Cinderella Ate My Daughter*. Now she writes about how young women navigate and negotiate being sexual today.

Websites

Adoption.com (www.adoption.com). This is an unbiased site for parents-to-be considering adoption.

Advocates for Youth (www.advocatesforyouth.org). This site approaches youth sexual health from a rights, respect, responsibility approach by providing lots of facts and chances to advocate for access to sexual health care and education. Advocates for Youth just released an amazing sexuality education program that's free to download. Take a look at it, or get your school to adopt the curriculum!

Bedsider (www.bedsider.org). The answer to any question about contraception can be found here! This site has a great tool that can help you choose the right method for you, and also has a national directory of health centers and emergency contraception access. Finally, it also has reminder features to help you remember to take your birth control!

The Guttmacher Institute (www.guttmacher.org). Heavy on the research, this website is great for school research or to get the most reliable information on what your state's policies are regarding access to sexual and reproductive health care.

Love Is Respect (www.loveisrespect.org). This site has lots of information about healthy and unhealthy relationships, plus quizzes you can take to learn more about your own relationship. It also has a text and hotline feature for those who need immediate help.

Palo Alto Medical Foundation (www.pamf.org/teen). Provides great health information for young people about many important health topics.

PFLAG (www.pflag.org). A great national organization that supports gay teens and those who care about them. Find a group in your area or maybe even start your own chapter!

RAINN (www.rainn.org). One of the most comprehensive sites on sexual abuse and rape. Accurate information along with a list of resources to get help and support.

Sex Etc. (www.sexetc.org). This website features stories written by young people, and fact-checked by health professionals, about sex and sexuality. It covers not only the facts, but also has a lot of interesting articles and opinions that are sure to spark some great thinking and possibly debate.

SexInfo Online (www.soc.ucsb.edu/sexinfo/category#TeenCorner). This site has a place to ask a sexpert a question, but you can also search its contents for great and well-researched information about sexual health and relationships. It's a pretty comprehensive site.

Sexuality and U (http://sexualityandu.ca/). Another great and comprehensive resource for all things related to sexuality and sexual health. It includes a birth control selection quiz and is run by the Society of Obstetricians and Gynae-cologists of Canada.

The Sexuality Information and Education Council of the United States (www.siecus.org). This site is run by a nonprofit whose goal is for everyone to have access to accurate information on sex and sexual health. It is a great resource for learning about sexuality education policies and advocacy.

The Trevor Project (www.trevorproject.org). Dedicated to helping LGBTQ youth who are feeling suicidal. It includes a text feature, hotline, and live chat on the site. People are there to help you.

Video Channels

Laci Green. Check out Laci Green's YouTube channel to get her take on all sorts of issues related to sexuality and relationships (I personally love her takes on labia and consent). She was named one of the thirty most influential people on the Internet by *Time* magazine! Note: Some of the language she uses may mean her videos are better suited for older youth.

Midwest Teen Sex Show. The Midwest Teen Sex Show video channel on YouTube was created by Nikol Hasler and covers all sorts of really taboo sexuality top-ics with a lot of humor and some good facts and advice.

Hotlines

Need someone to talk to? Check out these toll-free lines and call these people who can provide support. They are there because they want to help *you*.

Boys Town National Hotline (1-800-448-3000). For over twenty years, Boys Town has been helping young people of all genders with all sorts of issues. Its specialty is suicide prevention, but it can support you with a range of problems. If you don't feel like talking, you can go to http://www.yourlifey-ourvoice.org/ to get online chat or email services.

Child Help USA (1-800-422-4453). This is the National Child Abuse Hotline. If you believe you are experiencing some kind of abuse, please call this number from a safe location.

Love Is Respect (call 1-866-331-9474 or text "loveis" to 22522). If you believe you or a friend is in an abusive relationship, these people can help. Visit www.loveisrespect.org as well for live chat.

The National Hopeline Network (1-800-SUICIDE or 1-800-784-2433). The Hopeline will connect anyone who calls to the certified suicide crisis center nearest the caller's location anywhere in the United States.

National Runaway Safeline (1-800-RUNAWAY). A place to call 24/7 where people can listen, give support, and offer resources. Visit this website at http://www.1800runaway.org/ for a chat option as well.

National STD Hotline (1-800-CDC-INFO or 1-800-232-4636). Specialists provide health information about STDs at this hotline.

RAINN (1-800-656-HOPE [4673]). This hotline will automatically transfer you to the rape crisis center nearest you, anywhere in the United States.

The Trevor Project (1-866-488-7386). The Trevor Project provides crisis intervention, including suicide prevention, for LBGTQ youth. Visit this website at www.trevorproject.org for text and chat options as well.

Index

About the Author

L. Kris Gowen received her PhD in child and adolescent development from the Stanford School of Education and her EdM in human development and psychology from the Harvard Graduate School of Education. Since then, she has published several professional manuscripts on her research related to adolescence/young adulthood with foci on healthy relationships, mental health, sexuality education, and body image. Over the years, her advice for young people has appeared in magazines such as *Seventeen*, *Teen People*, and *Young and Modern* (where she served on the advisory board), and on several websites.

Gowen currently lives in Portland, Oregon, where she serves on the Oregon Youth Sexual Health Partnership and the advisory board of My Future, My Choice, a state-sponsored sexuality education program designed for sixth-grade students. She is also Senior Research Associate with the Evaluation Core at Oregon Health and Science University. She is an avid hockey fan and fancies herself a karaoke rock star.